Management of Patients with Traumatic Injuries

Editor

KAREN S. BERGMAN

CRITICAL CARE NURSING CLINICS OF NORTH AMERICA

www.ccnursing.theclinics.com

Consulting Editor
JAN FOSTER

June 2015 • Volume 27 • Number 2

ELSEVIER

1600 John F. Kennedy Boulevard • Suite 1800 • Philadelphia, Pennsylvania, 19103-2899

http://www.theclinics.com

CRITICAL CARE NURSING CLINICS OF NORTH AMERICA Volume 27, Number 2
June 2015 ISSN 0899-5885, ISBN-13: 978-0-323-38882-5

Editor: Kerry Holland
Developmental Editor: Colleen Viola

Critical Care Nursing Clinics of North America (ISSN 0899-5885) is published quarterly by Elsevier Inc., 360 Park Avenue South, New York, NY 10010-1710. Months of issue are March, June, September, and December. Business and Editorial Offices: 1600 John F. Kennedy Blvd., Suite 1800, Philadelphia, PA 19103-2899. Periodicals postage paid at New York, NY and additional mailing offices. Subscription prices are $150.00 per year for US individuals, $328.00 per year for US institutions, $80.00 per year for US students and residents, $200.00 per year for Canadian individuals, $412.00 per year for Canadian institutions, $230.00 per year for international individuals, $412.00 per year for international institutions and $115.00 per year for Canadian and international students/residents. To receive student/resident rate, orders must be accompanied by name of affiliated institution, data of term, and the *signature* of program/residency coordinator on institution letterhead. Orders will be billed at individual rate until proof of status is received. Foreign air speed delivery is included in all *Clinics* subscription prices. All prices are subject to change without notice. **POSTMASTER:** Send address changes to *Critical Care Nursing Clinics of North America*, Elsevier Health Sciences Division, Subscription Customer Service, 3251 Riverport Lane, Maryland Heights, MO 63043. **Customer Service: 1-800-654-2452 (US and Canada); 314-447-8871 (outside US and Canada). Fax: 314-447-8029. E-mail:** JournalsCustomerService-usa@elsevier.com **(for print support) and** JournalsOnlineSupport-usa@elsevier.com **(for online support).**

Reprints. For copies of 100 or more of articles in this publication, please contact the Commercial Reprints Department, Elsevier Inc., 360 Park Avenue South, New York, New York, 10010-1710; Tel.: 212-633-3874, Fax: 212-633-3820, and E-mail: reprints@elsevier.com.

Critical Care Nursing Clinics of North America is covered in *MEDLINE/PubMed (Index Medicus), International Nursing Index, Nursing Citation Index, Cumulative Index to Nursing and Allied Health Literature,* and *RNdex Top 100.*

Contributors

CONSULTING EDITOR

JAN FOSTER, PhD, APRN, CNS
Formerly, Associate Professor, College of Nursing, Texas Woman's University, Houston; Currently, President, Nursing Inquiry and Intervention Inc., The Woodlands, Texas

EDITOR

KAREN S. BERGMAN, PhD, RN, CNRN
Assistant Professor, Western Michigan University; Nurse Scientist, Bronson Methodist Hospital, Kalamazoo, Michigan

AUTHORS

VALERIE BEEKMANS, RN, BSN
Neuro Critical Care, Bronson Methodist Hospital, Kalamazoo, Michigan

KAREN S. BERGMAN, PhD, RN, CNRN
Assistant Professor, Western Michigan University; Nurse Scientist, Bronson Methodist Hospital, Kalamazoo, Michigan

ELIZABETH J. BRIDGES, PhD, RN, CCNS, FCCM, FAAN, Colonel USAFR NC (retired)
Associate Professor, Biobehavioral Nursing and Health Systems, University of Washington School of Nursing; Clinical Nurse Researcher, University of Washington Medical Center, Seattle, Washington

JENNIFER M. CARPENTER, MSN, RN, CPN
Clinical Instructor, Department of Education Services, Bronson Children's Hospital, Kalamazoo, Michigan

SAMARA A. CHAMPION, RN, CPN
Department of Pediatric Intensive Care Unit, Bronson Children's Hospital, Kalamazoo, Michigan

SCOTT B. DAVIDSON, MD, FACS
Medical Director, Trauma, Burn, and Surgical Critical Care Program, Trauma Surgery Services, Bronson Methodist Hospital, Kalamazoo, Michigan

SCOTT A. DRIESENGA, PhD
Psychology Service, VA Medical Center – Battle Creek, Battle Creek, Michigan

STEPHEN A. FIGUEROA, MD
Assistant Professor, Department of Neurology and Neurotherapeutics, UT Southwestern Medical Center, Dallas, Texas

LISA N. HEWITT, RN, MSN, APRN-BC, ACNP
Department of Trauma and Disaster Management, Parkland Hospital, Dallas, Texas

THUY-TIEN HO, PA
Department of Neurology and Neurotherapeutics, UT Southwestern Medical Center, Dallas, Texas

JENNIFER L. KENYON, RN
Pediatric Transport, Department of Pediatric Intensive Care Unit, Bronson Children's Hospital, Kalamazoo, Michigan

MARGARET A. LANDON, BSN, RN, CCRN
Department of Pediatric Intensive Care Unit, Bronson Children's Hospital, Kalamazoo, Michigan

RICHARD N. LESPERANCE, MD
Trauma and Acute Care Surgery Fellow, Division of Trauma and Surgical Critical Care, Vanderbilt University Medical Center, Nashville, Tennessee

KIM LITWACK, PhD, RN, FAAN, APNP
Associate Dean for Academic Affairs, University of Wisconsin-Milwaukee College of Nursing, Milwaukee, Wisconsin; Family Nurse Practitioner, Advanced Pain Management, Madison, Wisconsin

DOROTHY T. MACK, BAN, RN, CPN, CCRN, C-PNT
Pediatric Transport, Department of Pediatric Intensive Care Unit, Bronson Children's Hospital, Kalamazoo, Michigan

ZAKRAUS MAHDAVI, MD
Department of Neurology and Neurotherapeutics, UT Southwestern Medical Center, Dallas, Texas

CATHY A. MAXWELL, PhD, RN
Vanderbilt University School of Nursing, Nashville, Tennessee

MARGARET M. MCNEILL, PhD, RN, APRN-CNS, CCRN, CCNS, NE-BC, CIP, FAAN, Colonel USAF NC (retired)
Perianesthesia Clinical Nurse Specialist, Department of Professional and Clinical Development, Frederick Memorial Hospital, Frederick, Maryland

DONNA L. MOYER, PhD, RN, PCNS-BC
Clinical Nurse Specialist, Department of Nursing Professional Practice, Bronson Children's Hospital, Kalamazoo, Michigan

TIMOTHY C. NUNEZ, MD, FACS
Associate Professor, Department of Surgery, Tennessee Valley VA Medical Center, Nashville, Tennessee

DAIWAI M. OLSON, PhD, RN
Associate Professor, Department of Neurology and Neurotherapeutics, UT Southwestern Medical Center, Dallas, Texas

THOMAS PICARD, MD
Psychology Service, VA Medical Center – Battle Creek, Battle Creek, Michigan

NAREGNIA PIERRE-LOUIS, MD
Department of Neurology and Neurotherapeutics, UT Southwestern Medical Center, Dallas, Texas

JESSICA L. RODRIGUEZ, PhD
Psychology Service, VA Medical Center – Battle Creek, Battle Creek, Michigan

JEFF STROMSWOLD, RN, BSN, CCRN
Neuro Critical Care, Bronson Methodist Hospital, Kalamazoo, Michigan

SHERI L. VANDENBERG, BS, RN
Trauma Research Coordinator, Trauma Surgery Services, Bronson Methodist Hospital, Kalamazoo, Michigan

Contents

> Mass casualty incidents are events in which the number of injured patients exceeds the resources of the health care institution to the degree that care may not be available or may be limited for a portion of the casualties. Mass casualty incidents are increasing in frequency throughout the United States. Managing mass casualty incidents has not traditionally been part of the nursing curriculum; however, our changing world requires us to become educated and prepared to respond to these scenarios. This article focuses on intentional explosive disasters and the nursing and institutional response to these incidents. This information is of value to nursing professionals and other health care providers.

> Each year thousands of children are hospitalized for traumatic injuries associated with physical abuse. Nurses in the pediatric intensive care unit must be knowledgeable and skilled in caring for the physical, psychological, emotional, social, and developmental needs of such children and their families. This article provides direction for pediatric nurses working in the critical care setting. Specifically, it describes the nursing care of children in a pediatric intensive care unit where the mechanism of nonaccidental injury is blunt force to the head, abdomen, or musculoskeletal system, based on standards put forth by the American Association of Critical-Care Nurses.

> Injury in older adults is a looming public health crisis. This article provides a broad overview of geriatric trauma across the continuum of care. After a review of the epidemiology of geriatric trauma, optimal approaches to patient care are presented for triage and transport, trauma team activation and initial assessment, inpatient management, and injury prevention. Special emphasis is given to assessment of frailty, advanced care planning, and transitions of care.

Posttraumatic stress disorder (PTSD) can have a significant negative impact on the physical, emotional, and mental health of individuals. This article discusses the prevalence, risk factors, and diagnostic criteria for PTSD. Given the high incidence of PTSD in the Veteran population, much attention has been given to assessment and treatment issues. Treatment options for PTSD are discussed, including the 2 most effective treatments, prolonged exposure and cognitive processing therapy. Special issues concerning the treatment of Veterans are also reviewed.

Intimate partner violence (IPV) is a worldwide epidemic that has been prevalent in society since biblical times. IPV affects women long after the abuse stops, with victims of IPV having generalized worsening of health, including depression and increased thoughts of suicide and suicide attempts. It is not uncommon for victims of IPV to be killed by their partner. Through regular screening and education, clinicians can detect the violence before it is too late. Health care professionals have a unique opportunity to stop the cycle of abuse by intervening, promoting safety, and preventing the death of IPV victims.

Blast trauma can kill or injure by multiple different mechanisms, not all of which may be obvious on initial presentation. Patients injured by blast effects should be treated as having multisystem trauma and managed according to Advanced Trauma Life Support guidelines. For the most severely injured patients, damage control resuscitation should be practiced until definitive hemorrhage control has been achieved. Patients with blast injuries may present in mass-casualty episodes that can overwhelm local resources. This article reviews some specific injuries, as well as the importance of mild traumatic brain injury. The importance of rehabilitation is discussed.

Management of Patients with Traumatic Injuries

CRITICAL CARE NURSING
CLINICS OF NORTH AMERICA

Preface

The Complex Nature of Trauma

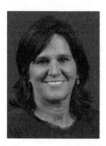

Karen S. Bergman, PhD, RN, CNRN
Editor

This issue of *Critical Care Nursing Clinics of North America* focuses on the complex nature of trauma. Care of the trauma patient involves understanding the intricate physiology of managing persons with multiple injuries. In addition to the physical injuries, persons often suffer from the psychological impact of trauma, which must also be addressed. Best practice for the management of the trauma patient is ever-changing, and this issue contains a series of articles to provide evidence-based information for the care of the trauma population across the life spectrum.

Trauma is a phenomenon that often occurs without warning, such as in the case of the Boston Marathon bombings or the attack on the World Trade Centers. When mass casualty trauma occurs, health care providers need to be prepared. Both civilian and military providers of trauma services must have a plan for the rapid influx of severely injured patients in just a moment's notice. Vandenberg and Davidson provide an excellent article on preparing for mass casualty incidents with information that can be applied to both smaller and larger trauma centers.

Special considerations often apply to trauma patients based on age. Moyer and colleagues provide evidence to support the care of the pediatric nonaccidental trauma patients and the unique nature of the child as a patient, along with the psychosocial aspects of caring for the child abuse patient and family. The majority of the articles in this issue focus on the adult patient, and Maxwell provides an excellent summary of care of the geriatric trauma patient and the special considerations that the elderly require.

Adequate resuscitation of a trauma patient is critical to survival and improved outcomes. Bridges and McNeill present a wealth of information on resuscitation and monitoring of the trauma patient for providing the optimal care. In addition to monitoring resuscitation efforts, this publication provides an update on advances in cerebral monitoring as well as strategies for neuroprotection in the brain-injured population.

All complex trauma cases require pain management. Pain management in the general population is complex, and caring for the trauma patient with potentially

Crit Care Nurs Clin N Am 27 (2015) xi–xii
http://dx.doi.org/10.1016/j.cnc.2015.03.001
0899-5885/15/$ – see front matter © 2015 Published by Elsevier Inc.

many co-occurring injuries can be even more difficult. This issue includes an excellent article on pain management in military trauma, which can also be applied to most civilian cases as well.

We round out this special issue of the *Critical Care Nursing Clinics of North America* with articles pertinent to many trauma patients, yet very unique in nature. Driesenga and colleagues present evidence-based treatments for posttraumatic stress disorder, a condition that exists but is often overlooked in the trauma population. Also included is an article on intimate partner violence, and the role of the health care provider in protecting patients. This article applies to all health care providers who need to be vigilant of signs of partner abuse and to know what to do to protect the patient. Because this issue is dedicated to trauma, violence, and war, it is important to include an article about the special considerations for blast injuries. Blasts are a mechanism of injury not frequently seen in civilian health care, but very common in military and mass casualty arenas, and this article provides information about identification and treatment of injuries to improve outcomes of trauma patients.

We hope that you find this special issue of *Critical Care Nursing Clinics of North America* helpful to your practice. Improving the care and outcomes of persons suffering from traumatic injury is the goal of all the authors in this issue, and their knowledge and expertise were essential for creating this publication for you.

Karen S. Bergman, PhD, RN, CNRN
Western Michigan University/
Bronson Methodist Hospital
601 John Street, Box 88
Kalamazoo, MI 49008, USA

E-mail address:
Bergmank@Bronsonhg.org

Preparation for Mass Casualty Incidents

Sheri L. VandenBerg, BS, RN[a],*, Scott B. Davidson, MD, FACS[b]

KEYWORDS

- Mass casualty incidents • Acts of terrorism • Disaster response • Explosions
- Blast injury

KEY POINTS

- In mass casualty incidents, the number of injured patients exceeds the resources of the health care institution; the goal of disaster medical care is to provide the greatest good for the greatest number of victims.
- The most experienced medical provider should be in charge of triaging victims and should reassess and retriage frequently, because the patient's conditions may deteriorate and hospital resources fluctuate.
- Unique blast injury patterns may include any combination of crush, burn, blunt, penetrating, and traumatic amputation.
- Damage control resuscitation involves balanced blood component transfusion and damage control surgery.

INTRODUCTION

It is a beautiful Saturday morning in October and by all appearances another busy day in the emergency department (ED) of your hospital. Fifty-five of the 70 beds in the ED are filled when an unusual call comes across your medical control telephone. An explosion at the farmer's market has just occurred and first responders are estimating 150 injured. As the ED charge nurse what is your first priority? What is your strategy for incoming victims and current patients already in your ED? Are you familiar with mass casualty triage? Are you knowledgeable about bomb and blast injury patterns, tourniquet use, and damage control resuscitation? Is there a plan for additional staff and how they can contribute to the response? How will your institution make available

Funding Sources: The authors have no sources of funding to disclose.
Conflict of Interest: The authors have no conflict of interest to disclose.
[a] Trauma Surgery Services, Bronson Methodist Hospital, 601 John Street, Box 67, Kalamazoo, MI 49007, USA; [b] Trauma, Burn, and Surgical Critical Care Program, Trauma Surgery Services, Bronson Methodist Hospital, 601 John Street, Box 67, Kalamazoo, MI 49007, USA
* Corresponding author.
E-mail address: vandensh@bronsonhg.org

Crit Care Nurs Clin N Am 27 (2015) 157–166
http://dx.doi.org/10.1016/j.cnc.2015.02.008
0899-5885/15/$ – see front matter © 2015 Elsevier Inc. All rights reserved.

essential critical care beds or create alternative sites? Can you accommodate the swarm of family and media about to invade your institution? Are you familiar with post-event debriefing and analysis? These are some of the challenges that a mass casualty incident (MCI) presents, and as a nurse you will be indispensable in the response. Managing MCIs has not traditionally been part of the nursing curriculum; however, the changing world we live in requires us to become educated and prepared to respond to these scenarios.[1] This article focuses on the nurse's role in MCIs as a result of explosive acts of terrorism.

DISASTER DEFINITION

MCIs are events where the number of injured patients exceeds the resources of the health care institution to the degree that care may not be available or may be limited for a portion of the casualties.[2,3] Multiple casualty incidents are different in that the hospital is able to respond to a surge in their capacity, which strains but does not over-whelm a facility's resources.[2,4] MCIs may be the result of a natural disaster, such as those caused by weather and the environment, or they may be man-made including unintentional and intentional events (**Table 1**). Intentional disasters are considered terrorism and may involve weapons or bombs that have the ability to produce large numbers of casualties that can easily challenge a health care system. The mass shoot-ings at Columbine High School in Littleton, Colorado, at Sandy Hook Elementary School in Connecticut, and at the movie theater in Aurora, Colorado along with the bombings in Oklahoma City and at the 2013 Boston Marathon serve to remind us that these types of terrorist attacks are increasing in frequency in the United States.

PRINCIPALS OF DISASTER MANAGEMENT

Although types of disasters vary, the health care response includes basic elements that are applicable in all disasters (**Box 1**). The incident command system (ICS) is the initial standard element in disaster response. The roles assigned within the ICS should be based on functional requirements, not titles or politics. The ICS should be flexible and scalable for use in any type or size MCI.[3] The ability to manage a surge of injured patients relies on well trained and drilled responders rather than readily avail-able volunteers. Nursing and medical care rendered in an MCI is much different than conventional care, with the emphasis on doing the greatest good for the greatest num-ber of victims.[1,3,5–7] Caution must be exercised to optimize the use of critical resources.[8]

Table 1 Types of disasters		
Natural	**Man-Made Unintentional**	**Man-Made Intentional**
Hurricanes	Plane crash	Arson
Floods	Train crash	Biologic agents
Tornadoes	Multicar crash	Chemical agents
Landslides	Gas leak/explosion	Radioactive agents
Volcanoes		Explosions/bombs
Earthquakes		Active shooter
Tsunamis		
Severe weather		

> **Box 1**
> **Key points of MCI management**
>
> - Disaster management teams are based on functional roles, not titles
> - Medical care in an MCI is different than conventional care
> - Goal of disaster medical care is the greatest good for the greatest number of victims

DISASTER PREPARATION

Planning, practice, and debriefing are essential to meet the demands an MCI places on a health care facility and community.[3,9–12] Because of the frequency in which they respond to MCIs, the US military has developed standardized response protocols,[2,13–16] as has Israel, which relies on national standard templates.[5,6,11,17] It may be helpful to refer to these sources as proved evidence-based practice when formulating your institution's disaster management plan. Planning is the first step in developing an infrastructure that provides the necessary personnel, supplies, equipment, and support to meet the demands of an MCI that presents to your institution. Preparation must also extend to the surrounding community and involve interagency planning. Table top discussions alone are not adequate.[4,6,7,18,19]

DISASTER DRILLS

Practical, real-life, hands-on mass casualty drills using your institutional disaster response plan, and community-wide drills are essential for an integrated response to an MCI.[5,6,9,20] Only in physically walking through mock scenarios and treating simulated patients can deficiencies or problems with the disaster response plan become evident. Debriefing gives you the opportunity to identify those areas and formulate solutions before an MCI. One of the most consistent messages cited following the Boston Marathon bombings was the crucial role planning and participation in routine hospital, city, and state-wide drills were in preparing the Boston hospital community. This helped to facilitate an immediate response in a calm and confident manner despite the surrounding chaos.[21–25]

DISASTER RESPONSE

From the moment your institution is notified of an MCI in which you will be receiving victims, a checklist of tasks specific to your hospital disaster management plan should be followed (**Box 2**). The ED is the center of the response[26] with the charge nurse fulfilling an essential role. Trauma and operating room (OR) personnel should report to

> **Box 2**
> **Initial management checklist**
>
> - Clear ED
> - Establish incident commander
> - Qualified staff report to ED
> - Create critical care beds
> - Hold OR and radiology nonemergent procedures

the ED as soon as possible. Patients currently in the ED need to be transferred to inpatient beds if they cannot be discharged. All inpatients that are able should be discharged as soon as possible and postanesthesia patients should be held in postanesthesia care unit instead of transferring to inpatient beds.[7,9] Ongoing procedures in the OR and radiology department should continue but all nonemergent procedures should be postponed. Transferring current critical care patients as able to medical beds makes available that critically necessary resource.[5] Specialty units, such as cardiac catheterization, outpatient surgery, endoscopy suites, and chest pain observation units, may prove to be the simplest to transform into temporary critical care beds. Adapting the remainder of beds to meet the needs the MCI presents may include converting single rooms to doubles.[7] Nursing staff should be called in from home and shifts should overlap because nursing availability is the key restriction to the number of injured an institution can accommodate in an MCI.[6,7] Flexibility in duties is essential; however, ED and critical care nurses are not interchangeable with floor nurses, and staff that does not usually treat trauma and critical care patients is not qualified to do so now.[6,7,26,27]

SECURITY

The perimeter of your institution and especially the ED needs to be secured. Expect the presence and involvement of local, state, and federal authorities as the event unfolds. Be aware that your site may be vulnerable to possible secondary attacks and hostile patients, including the possibility that the perpetrators could be among the injured.

MASS CASUALTY INCIDENT VOLUME

The number of patients arriving at your institution depends on the density of people on the scene, the number of attackers or bombs, and type and size of explosives or ammunition used (**Box 3**). Consider the circumstances of the incident; multiple or single shooter, car bomb or suicide bombing, open air or enclosed space explosion?[6,28] These facts should help in estimating the number of injured you could receive. Anticipate a flood of families and/or friends descending on your hospital looking for injured loved ones. Establish a large information center to help families and friends locate their loved one and receive status updates in a location removed from the ED.[6] Nurses serve a valuable resource in explaining a patient's condition and necessary treatment. Pictures of the victims using Polaroid film/cameras or digital cameras facilitate patient identification.[29] Social workers and psychologists also provide valuable support to families in this area. Ideally an area with computer access and good cell phone reception should be designated as the family information center.[6]

Box 3
Severity by the numbers

20%, victims with severe injuries

30%, victims with moderate injuries

50%, victims with mild injuries

Data from Lynn M, Gurr D, Memon A, et al. Management of conventional mass casualty incidents: ten commandments for hospital planning. J Burn Care Res 2006;27:649–58.

COMMUNICATION

Be prepared for a challenging communication environment. Cellular phone networks can be shut down either by overload or by law enforcement for fear of a cell phone activating secondary explosive devices.[10] Portable two-way radios, megaphones, and identification vests for staff with assignments printed on them are helpful in aiding in communication amid the confusion of a mass casualty event.[6] One of the most frequently cited barriers in debriefings following actual mass casualty events has been poor communication, along with confusion and a lack of command or control.[6–10,20]

TRIAGE

Prioritizing the injured in an MCI is different from conventional triage, and occurs in the prehospital and hospital setting, perhaps multiple times.[3] Although conventional triage focuses on the greatest good for the individual patient, disaster triage focuses on the greatest good for the greatest number of patients (**Box 4**). The objective of triage in an MCI is to quickly identify the most critical patients with the greatest chance of survival using minimal resources and time. The most experienced medical person with knowledge of the consequences of burn, blast, crush, and amputation injuries should be designated to rapidly categorize the victims into the appropriate levels of care.[3,5,7,8,11,26]

FIELD TRIAGE

Initial triage at the scene of an MCI may consist of quick categorization of victims where they lay using color coding with red for acute and green for nonacute. Tagging victims is helpful if available on scene or alternatively writing red or green on their forehead in the absence of tags. It may be beneficial to have victims who can walk (nonacute/green) ambulate to a designated area nearby separating the ambulatory from nonambulatory wounded.[3] Although victims who did not survive on the scene need to be transported to the morgue, their transfer may be delayed to preserve transportation resources. Expectant patients who are severely wounded and unlikely to survive are also delayed. Care may be provided if resources allow for these victims after those who are deemed most likely to survive have been treated.[3,5,8,11,26]

HOSPITAL TRIAGE

The medical person most experienced with the type and severity of injuries unique to the MCI should be in charge of prioritizing victims on arrival to your ED, most likely a trauma surgeon. Rapid categorization and color labeling is based on the level of care victims require from injuries sustained, the likelihood of survival, and available resources (**Fig. 1**).[3,5,28]

Box 4
Triage considerations

- Severity of injury
- Likelihood of survival
- Available resources

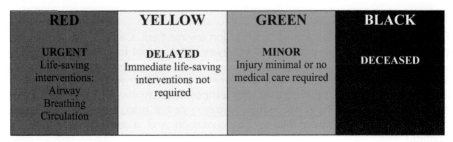

RED	YELLOW	GREEN	BLACK
URGENT Life-saving interventions: Airway Breathing Circulation	DELAYED Immediate life-saving interventions not required	MINOR Injury minimal or no medical care required	DECEASED

Fig. 1. Medical triage.

Avoid undertriage, which delays treatment for a critically injured patient, and overtriage, which assigns noncritical patients to immediate care and may exhaust limited resources. Re-evaluate patient status frequently because their condition may rapidly change necessitating a different designation or level of care. While casualties are still arriving, minimally acceptable care is given to preserve resources until the scope of the MCI and volumes are known.[26] Use a simple documentation system that does not depend on power supply.[19] Writing with permanent marker on the patient if necessary ensures each subsequent care provider knows what has been done and given. Eventually a balance is reached when there are no more incoming wounded and there is adequate staff, space, and supplies to manage the remainder of the MCI.[4]

BLAST INJURY

Victims of blast injury present a complex diagnostic and treatment challenge. Care providers may encounter patients with any combination of blunt, penetrating, and/or burn injuries; not a common scenario for most civilian hospitals (**Fig. 2**). Blast injuries are classified into four categories, with the possibility to have one or multiple levels of injury (**Box 5**). Primary blast injury is a result of the overpressurization force (blast wave) impacting the body surface. Likely injuries include tympanic membrane rupture (compromised hearing), pulmonary damage (blast lung injury), air embolism, and hollow viscus injury.

Secondary blast injury results from flying debris and bomb fragments or projectiles often placed to maximize injury, such as nails, ball bearings, and screws. This causes

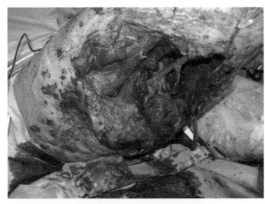

Fig. 2. Blast injury to right posterior thigh from suicide bomb in Iraq. (*Courtesy of* Lt. Col. Scott B. Davidson, MD, FACS.)

Box 5
Blast injury categories

- Primary blast injury: caused by pressure of blast wave
- Secondary blast injury: struck by flying debris and bomb fragments
- Tertiary blast injury: propelled by blast wave into stationary object
- Quaternary blast injury: thermal burns; inhalation of dust, smoke, and chemicals; crush injuries

---

penetrating trauma, which may not be obvious, but is revealed on radiologic evaluation. Also expect fragmentation injuries and blunt trauma with secondary blast injury. Tertiary blast injury is a result of the victim being thrown by the blast wind and impacting a stationary object. Common injuries include blunt and penetrating trauma, fractures, and traumatic amputations. Quaternary blast injury encompasses all other injuries sustained in the blast including chemical and thermal burns, asphyxia, toxic exposures, and exacerbations of chronic illnesses.[3,5,28,30] Nurses are called on to assist physicians with these very complex wounds. However, the treatment algorithm as outlined in advanced trauma life support remains the same; airway, breathing, and circulation are still the focus of initial care. Interventions are likely brief with re-evaluation and retriage mandatory.

CRUSH INJURY

Crush injury and crush syndrome may result from structural collapse after a bombing or explosion. Crush injury is defined as compression of extremities or other parts of the body that causes muscle swelling and/or neurologic disturbance in the affected body area. Crush syndrome consists of localized crush injury with systemic manifestations. Most importantly, traumatic rhabdomyolysis (muscle breakdown) releases toxic substances into the bloodstream that can result in local tissue injury, organ dysfunction (renal failure), and metabolic abnormalities. Treatment is centered on preventing renal failure with aggressive fluid hydration, with a goal of obtaining a urine output of 200 to 300 mL/h. Mannitol and bicarbonate may be used at the discretion of the treating physician.[30]

EXTREMITY INJURY

Soft tissue and musculoskeletal systems have the highest incidence of bodily injury in survivors of bombings (**Fig. 3**). Traumatic amputations are reported in 1% to 3% of blast victims.[30] Initial care for active hemorrhage is direct pressure with the application of a pressure dressing. If direct pressure is not successful, tourniquet application or operative intervention is required. Patients may present with formal tourniquets in place or improvised tourniquets placed by bystanders. Properly placed tourniquets should be at least 1.5-in wide and placed just proximal to the bleeding point. The time applied should be recorded on the tourniquet, because total tourniquet time should not exceed 2 hours. Tourniquets should only be removed by physicians prepared to handle life- or limb-threatening bleeding. Continued nursing observation and assessment of the victim is crucial to the treating physician and may impact the order in which patients proceed to the OR.

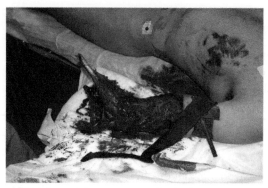

Fig. 3. Traumatic amputation with tourniquet applied. (*Courtesy of* Lt. Col. Scott B. Davidson, MD, FACS.)

RESOURCE USE

Nurses are valuable contributors in the planning and execution of their institution's response. Knowledge of the rate-limiting factors as they pertain to the care of mass casualty patients aids institutions and incident commanders as to their resource capabilities and guides them in decisions to transfer or divert patients if possible. Triage decisions may also be profoundly affected as supplies run low or are exhausted.

TRANSFUSION REQUIREMENTS

The conflicts in Afghanistan and Iraq have changed the algorithm in how surgeons resuscitate critically injured patients, specifically those that present in hemorrhagic shock or those at high risk of going into shock. There are two stages in this new era of damage control resuscitation (DCR): transfusion of balanced ratios of blood components and limited crytalloid infusion, and damage control surgery.

Current data support a balanced blood component infusion of fresh frozen plasma (FFF), packed red blood cells (PRBC), and platelets in a 1:1:1 ratio.[15,16] It should be noted that not all patients require this regimen; it is at the discretion of the trauma surgeon or emergency physician and may also depend on the availability of blood products.

A study by Propper and colleagues[2] conducted at a US military hospital in Iraq involving 50 victims in three separate explosive mass casualty events examined specific resource use for these critically injured patients. Blood transfusions were required by 48% of all casualties with an average of 3.5 and 3.8 units of PRBC and FFF per patient, respectively. This requirement may be lower in civilian hospitals that are more likely to receive a higher percentage of less critically injured patients than the military hospitals because of a difference in triage and transfer criteria.[2]

OPERATING ROOM USE

Damage control surgery, the second stage of DCR may be used during an MCI. This strategy involves an initial abbreviated operation with the main goals being major hemorrhage control, eliminating sources of contamination, and temporary abdominal closure with subsequent transfer to a critical care unit. In the study by Propper and co-workers,[2] 76% of the blast victims required surgery with a mean OR time of 2.5 hours per patient. Nursing care and judgment are indispensable at this stage of resuscitation as the patient transitions from the OR to the critical care unit. Monitoring and treatment of acidosis, hypothermia, and coagulopathy are essential. Patients are returned to the OR in the ensuing 24 to 48 hours for definitive procedures and possible closures. Damage control procedures may also be performed by orthopedic and vascular surgeons.

Propper and coworkers[2] also describe the concept of parallel operating during an MCI whereby multiple surgical specialties operate simultaneously, including trauma surgery, orthopedic, and neurosurgery.[2] This allows for shorter OR times in critical patients and also establishes efficient use of OR resources to accommodate more casualties. This strategy is reliant on the superb skills of OR nurses in coordination and care.

DEBRIEFING

An MCI is an extraordinary event that will likely affect all aspects of hospital function. To help restore equilibrium to the institution, debriefings need to occur on many levels.[9,17,19,28,31] In analyzing the crisis and response, nurses are uniquely positioned with their clinical knowledge and understanding of administrative functions to participate in this evaluation. They may be called on to assess use of resources, evaluate patient flow and treatment, identify symptoms of posttraumatic stress disorder, and formulate strategies that may benefit their institution or others in future MCIs.

SUMMARY

There is no substitute for preparation. MCIs, although statistically rare, remain a real threat. Those in the health care profession must be vigilant in their own personal preparation for these possibilities. They must participate in and encourage their own institutions to plan, prepare, and practice for these potentially catastrophic events. Knowledge of triage, injury patterns, logistical challenges, and new paradigms in resuscitation aid in providing the greatest good for the greatest number.

REFERENCES

1. Krutz A, Olchin L. Nurses as first responders in a mass casualty: are you prepared? J Trauma Nurs 2012;19:122–9.
2. Propper BW, Rasmussen TE, Davidson SB, et al. Surgical response to multiple casualty incidents following single explosive events. J Trauma 2009;250:311–5.
3. Briggs SM. Advanced disaster medical response manual for providers. 2nd edition. Woodbury (CT): Cine'-Med Publishing; 2014.
4. Kearns RD, Cairns BA, Cairns CB. Surge capacity and capability. a review of the history and where the science is today regarding surge capacity during a mass casualty disaster. Front Public Health 2014;2:1–4.
5. Almogy G, Rivkind A. Surgical lessons learned from suicide bombing attacks. J Am Coll Surg 2006;202:313–9.
6. Lynn M, Gurr D, Memon A, et al. Management of conventional mass casualty incidents: ten commandments for hospital planning. J Burn Care Res 2006;27: 649–58.
7. Hick JL, Hanfling D, Burstein JL, et al. Health care facility and community strategies for patient care surge capacity. Ann Emerg Med 2004;44:253–61.
8. Committee on Trauma, American College of Surgeons. Disaster planning and management. In: Resources for the optimal care of the injured patient 2014, 6th edition. p. 149–54. Available at: http://www.facs.org/quality%20programs/trauma. Accessed November 20, 2014.

9. Erickson JI. A chief nurse's reflections on marathon Monday 2013. J Nurs Adm 2013;43:429–30.
10. Augustine JJ. What's in your all-hazards plan? In Boston they were prepared. Are you? EMS World 2013;42:18, 20, 23.
11. Einav S, Aharonson-Daniel L, Weissman C, et al. In-hospital resource utilization during multiple casualty incidents. Ann Surg 2006;243:533–40.
12. Frykberg ER, Tepas JJ. Terrorist bombings. Lessons learned from Belfast to Beirut. Ann Surg 1988;208:569–76.
13. Elster EA, Butler FK, Rasmussen TE. Implications of combat casualty care for mass casualty events. JAMA 2013;310:475–6.
14. Raja AS, Propper BW, VandenBerg SL, et al. Imaging utilization during explosive multiple casualty incidents. J Trauma 2010;68:1421–4.
15. Borgman MA, Spinella PC, Perkins JG, et al. The ratio of blood products transfused affects mortality in patients receiving massive transfusions at a combat support hospital. J Trauma 2007;63:805–13.
16. U.S. Army Institute of Surgical Care website. Available at: http://www.usair. amedd.army.mil. Accessed November 3, 2014.
17. Adini B, Peleg K. On constant alert: lessons to be learned from Israel's emergency response to mass-casualty terrorism incidents. Health Aff 2013;32:2179–85.
18. Kreimer S. The lessons of 9/11: nurses now better prepared for mass casualties. In: Nursezone.com. Available at: http://www.nursezone.com. Accessed July 21, 2014.
19. Richardson S, Ardagh M, Grainger P, et al. A moment in time: emergency nurses and the Canterbury earthquakes. Int Nurs Rev 2013;60:188–95.
20. Sloan HM. Responding to a multiple-casualty incident: room for improvement. J Emerg Nurs 2011;37:484–6.
21. Gebhardt MC. Patriots' day at the Boston marathon. Clin Orthop Relat Res 2013; 471:2045–6.
22. Biddinger PD, Baggish A, Harrington L, et al. Be prepared-the Boston marathon and mass-casualty events. N Engl J Med 2013;368:1958–60.
23. Kellermann AL, Peleg K. Lessons from Boston. N Engl J Med 2013;368:1956–7.
24. Eggertson L. Canadian doctor led bombing response at a Boston hospital. CMAJ 2013;185:E373–4.
25. Bluman EM. Boston marathon bombing. Foot Ankle Int 2013;34:1053–4.
26. Hirshberg A, Holcomb JB, Mattox KL. Hospital trauma care in multiple-casualty incidents: a critical view. Ann Emerg Med 2001;37:647–52.
27. Jagim J. Emergency preparedness response: building infrastructure. J Emerg Nurs 2007;33:567–70.
28. Almogy G, Belzberg H, Mintz Y, et al. Suicide bombing attacks. Updates and modifications to the protocol. Ann Surg 2004;239:295–303.
29. Liebergall MH, Braverman N, Shapira SC, et al. Role of nurses in a university hospital during mass casualty events. Am J Crit Care 2007;16:480–4.
30. Centers for Disease Control and Prevention. Blast injuries. Essential facts. Available at: http://emergency.cdc.gov/BlastInjuries. Accessed November 7, 2014.
31. Romer C, Hebda T. Disaster preparedness for bedside nurses-part three. In: Advance Healthcare Network for Nurses 2013. Available at: http://nursing. advanceweb.com. Accessed October 6, 2014.

Nonaccidental Trauma

Guidance for Nurses in the Pediatric Intensive Care Unit

Donna L. Moyer, PhD, RN, PCNS-BC[a],*,
Jennifer M. Carpenter, MSN, RN, CPN[b],
Margaret A. Landon, BSN, RN, CCRN[c],
Dorothy T. Mack, BAN, RN, CPN, CCRN, C-PNT[c], Jennifer L. Kenyon, RN[c],
Samara A. Champion, RN, CPN[c]

KEYWORDS

- Nonaccidental trauma • Physical abuse • Child abuse • Critical care
- Critical care nursing • Pediatric nursing

KEY POINTS

- Each year thousands of children are hospitalized for traumatic injuries associated with nonaccidental trauma and physical abuse.
- Nurses in the pediatric intensive care unit must be knowledgeable and skilled in caring for the physical, psychological, emotional, social, and developmental needs of physically abused children and their families.
- Nurses in an intensive care setting play an important role in maximizing health outcomes and minimizing the negative consequence of abuse for children and their families.

Nursing is the protection, promotion, and optimization of health and abilities, prevention of illness and injury, alleviation of suffering through the diagnosis and treatment of human response, and advocacy in the care of individuals, families, communities, and populations.
　　　　　　　　　　　　　　　　　　　　　　　　　—American Nurses Association

INTRODUCTION

Over 650,000 children in the United States are subject to physical, sexual, or emotional maltreatment and neglect each year.[1] Of these, approximately 4500 require

The authors have nothing to disclose.
[a] Department of Nursing Professional Practice, Bronson Children's Hospital, 601 John Street, Kalamazoo, MI 49007, USA; [b] Department of Education Services, Bronson Children's Hospital, 601 John Street, Kalamazoo, MI 49007, USA; [c] Department of Pediatric Intensive Care Unit, Bronson Children's Hospital, 601 John Street, Kalamazoo, MI 49007, USA
* Corresponding author. Bronson Children's Hospital, 601 John Street, Kalamazoo, MI 49007.
E-mail address: moyerd@bronsonhg.org

hospitalization for abusive injury.[2,3] The pervasive nature of child abuse makes it likely that all nurses who care for children in an acute care setting will encounter survivors of maltreatment. Yet many feel unprepared to provide care for this complex and vulnerable population.[4,5]

A child who is critically injured by abusive trauma needs nurses who are knowledgeable and skilled in addressing a wide range of physical, psychological, emotional, social, and developmental needs. Physical injuries are not managed in isolation, and nurses must be prepared to care for the whole of the child and family. Despite the advanced level of nursing care required, nurses rarely receive formal education on the matter and find little guidance in the literature. There is growing evidence related to the public health and medical particulars of maltreatment, including its incidence, identification, diagnosis, reporting, long-term sequelae, and prevention.[6] This literature contributes to nurses' basic understanding of child maltreatment but is of less value to directing bedside care in an intensive care unit. In fact, there is surprisingly little published information to guide nursing practice during the acute care phase of nonaccidental injury.[7,8]

This article provides direction for pediatric nurses in a critical care setting. Specifically, this article describes the nursing care of children in a pediatric intensive care unit where the mechanism of nonaccidental injury is blunt force to the head, abdomen, or musculoskeletal system, based on standards put forth by the American Association of Critical-Care Nurses (AACN).[9]

SIGNIFICANCE

The US Department of Health and Human Services publishes an annual report that describes the state of child abuse and neglect, as reported by child protective agencies. In its most recent report, an estimated 686,000 boys and girls younger than 18 years experience abuse or neglect.[1] Physical abuse accounts for nearly 20% of child maltreatment cases, where infants and young children are disproportionately affected. Infants younger than 1 year are most frequently involved, representing 13% of all victims. Children between ages 1 and 3 years account for an additional 21%, demonstrating that nearly one-third of abused and neglected children are younger than 3 years.[1] Among older children, there is increased risk for those with physical, intellectual, emotional, or other disabilities.[1,10,11]

Of all children who are physically abused, approximately 1.5% are hospitalized for related injuries.[3] Consistent with higher rates of maltreatment and injury severity, infants younger than 1 year are most frequently hospitalized.[2,3,10] Socioeconomic status and income also seem to be relevant factors in children's rates of hospitalization for abuse.[2,3]

Perpetrators

Across all forms of abuse and neglect, parents are the most frequent abusers (80%).[1] Children are maltreated by a nonparents in only 16% of abuse and neglect cases.[1] In cases where infants and children sustain fatal injuries, parents are again the most frequent offenders (80%). Biological mothers are the most frequent perpetrators of fatal abusive injury, followed by both parents together, and then by fathers.[1] Fatal injuries are caused by nonparents in 14% of cases.[1]

Long-Term Implications

For those who survive abusive trauma, the effects often persist beyond childhood. There is a strong association between abuse and physical, psychological, and behavioral health deficits later in life.[12–14] The severity, nature, and mechanism of a child's injury influence long-term outcome,[15,16] particularly with respect to continued physical deficit. It has been recognized, however, that a child's subjective sense of harm or threat is as important as actual injury severity in the development of psycho-emotional disability (**Box 1**).

Fatal Injury

With regard to abuse-related mortality, boys have a higher rate of fatal injury than girls.[1] In 2012, 1640 children died of abuse and neglect. Of those who died, 44% were physically abused.[1] The youngest children, while most vulnerable to maltreatment, also have high rates of associated mortality.[1,10] Almost 70% of abused or neglected children who died in 2012 were younger than 3 years.[10]

NONACCIDENTAL TRAUMA CAUSED BY BLUNT FORCE

Abuse is often recurrent among maltreated children.[1,24] It is important, therefore, for nurses to recognize injuries that are consistent with an abusive mechanism. The number of abusive injuries inflicted by blunt force has not been reported in the literature. Blunt force injury is a frequently recognized mechanism of injury, however, in abusive head trauma (AHT), visceral or abdominal trauma, and musculoskeletal injury. Nurses can improve recognition of physical abuse by better understanding unique characteristics of these injuries. By recognizing features of nonaccidental trauma, nurses can identify and report suspicious cases, so that social service agencies and legal action can ensure a child's future safety. Nurses are required by law in most states to report suspicion of child abuse to state agencies.[25]

Characteristics of Abusive Head Trauma

AHT is defined as "an injury to the skull or intracranial contents of an infant or young child due to inflicted blunt force and/or violent shaking."[26(p10)] AHT is preferred to shaken baby syndrome because the term is more inclusive. In a vast number of cases of AHT, the exact mechanism of injury may be unknown and a combination of blunt force and shaking might both contribute to eventual injury.[27]

AHT is a common type of nonaccidental injury, and one that frequently results in hospital admission.[3] The rate of AHT for infants younger than 1 year is 20 to 30 per 100,000 infants in the general population.[26] Approximately 25% to 30% of children younger than 2 years who have head trauma are injured by a nonaccidental cause.[27]

Box 1
Psychological dysfunction associated with nonaccidental trauma

- Posttraumatic stress disorder[17–20]
- Anxiety[15]
- Depression[15]
- Decreased life satisfaction[15]
- Suicidal ideation/suicide attempts[21,22]
- Eating disorders[21,23]
- Smoking and alcohol use[13,15,21]

Data from Refs.[13,15,17–23]

AHT generally results in more severe injury than accidental head trauma.[28] AHT is a leading cause of abuse-related morbidity and mortality[29,30] and results in greater lengths of stay and higher costs to treat than head injury due to accident.[28] Infants and children with AHT also demonstrate poorer outcomes and are less likely to survive until hospital discharge.[28,31] Low Glasgow Coma Scale scores, retinal and intraparenchymal hemorrhage, and cerebral edema are associated with mortality in AHT.[32] Those who survive frequently have permanent disability, persistent neurologic symptoms, and sensorimotor deficit.[33–35]

Because young children often cannot provide an account of the injury, and caregivers may be unaware or reticent to share the story, the exact mechanism of injury is often unknown during initial phases of care.[31,36] Infants present with a host of nonspecific symptoms, which may include apnea, seizures, lethargy, irritability, poor feeding, vomiting, listlessness, poor head control, and failure to track or focus.[29,31,37] Coupled with treatment delay, a vague history, changing accounts of an incident, or description of an accident that is inconsistent with the degree of physical injury, these findings warrant high suspicion for AHT.[7,37]

AHT may be associated with other physical injuries such as skull fractures, retinal hemorrhage, long bone fractures, metaphyseal fractures, rib fractures, and bruising.[38,39] The concurrent presence of rib fractures on radiologic examination or hematocrit less than 30 g/dL or platelet count greater than 400,000 platelets/mL should also raise suspicion for abuse.[31,40]

Characteristics of Abusive Abdominal Trauma

Abusive abdominal trauma (AAT) is a less common type of nonaccidental injury, but it is associated with poor outcomes and high rates of mortality.[41,42] It has been reported that the incidence of AAT is approximately 5 per million in children younger than 9 years, accounting for 3.8% to 4.3 % of hospital admissions for abuse.[43] Like other types of child maltreatment, AAT is most common in infants and young children.[43]

There are several anatomic differences that make children more susceptible to abdominal traumatic injury than adults, including weaker abdominal muscles, a shorter distance between the abdominal wall and vertebral column, and organs that extend beyond the rib cage.[44] Injury often results from direct blows to the abdomen or rapid deceleration.[45] The most common AAT injuries are to hollow organs and the liver, kidneys, and pancreas.[43,46] Cardiac injury is rare but should be considered in cases of thoracic trauma.[47]

Children with abusive abdominal injuries initially present with symptoms such as pain, vomiting, and signs of developing shock.[42] Abdominal tenderness, distension, and bruising may also be present.[45] Almost 2% of all children with nonaccidental injuries have been reported to have occult abdominal injury. Laboratory analysis to detect elevation of levels of liver and pancreatic enzymes, in addition to screening for occult blood in the child's urine and stool, is used to screen for less-obvious abdominal injury.[48] Concealment of inflicted trauma often contributes to delayed diagnosis and treatment.[42] Children can present, therefore, with progressing or advanced stages of peritonitis, sepsis, or shock.

Characteristics of Abusive Musculoskeletal Trauma

Fractures are a common injury associated with physical abuse.[49] Fractures result from either direct blow to the bone or shaking, twisting, pulling, pushing, or otherwise manipulating a child's limbs.[50] The incidence of abusive fractures is approximately 15 in 100,000 in children younger than 3 years and 36 in 100,000 in infants younger than 1 year.[51] Fractures are identified in up to one-third of children who have been physically abused.[52] Like other forms of abusive trauma, fractures occur more often in younger children.[49,53]

The femur, tibia, and humerus are the most frequently injured long bones in cases of abuse.[50] Infants and children with abusive fractures often present with pain, swelling, bone deformity, limited range of motion, altered function, or inability to bear weight.[50] With related treatment delay, missing explanation for injury, or history that is incompatible with the child's developmental age, suspicion for abuse is warranted.[50] The presence of multiple fractures, rib fractures, skull fractures, and any fracture in a non-ambulatory child also raise suspicion.[52]

Fractures, however, are also a common accidental childhood injury leading nurses to misattribute abusive fractures to mishap.[54] It has been demonstrated that 20% of abusive fractures are missed in health care visits,[55] particularly in boys, in whom accidental musculoskeletal injury is common. Delayed diagnosis, therefore, is common.

NURSING CARE IN THE PEDIATRIC INTENSIVE CARE UNIT

The AACN has published a set of standards, and related measurement criteria, for nurses who practice in critical care settings.[9] The standards are based on the nursing process and include general expectations related to assessment, diagnosis, outcomes identification, planning, implementation, and evaluation. The standards provide a framework on which to organize care for children who are hospitalized for nonaccidental injury.

American Association of Critical-Care Nurses Standard 1: Assessment

The nurse caring for the acutely and critically ill patient collects relevant data pertinent to the patient's health or situation.[9]

Initial impression
A tiered, systematic approach is used in the initial assessment of any child with traumatic injury.[56] An orderly and organized process of assessment yields reliable data based on which important clinical decisions can be made. The nurse begins by forming an initial impression of the child's condition. This brief initial assessment is complete within moments of seeing the child and is based on 3 assessment parameters: level of consciousness, work of breathing, and color.[56] The goal of the initial impression is to quickly identify life-threatening conditions, so that resuscitation can be promptly initiated. The mechanism of injury is largely irrelevant at this point.

Primary assessment
After the nurse forms an initial impression of the child's condition, and life-saving measures are initiated, a primary assessment is completed.[56] A primary assessment includes rapid evaluation of the child's airway, breathing, circulation, neurologic function, and exposure. The goal here is to identify the severity of the child's condition and direct further intervention. It is during the primary assessment that physical signs of abusive injury, such as bruising or overt fractures, may first be identified.[56] As urgent needs are identified in the primary assessment, they are addressed in an effort to stabilize the child's condition.

Secondary assessment
After the child's condition is stable, a more comprehensive evaluation is completed in secondary assessment.[56] A head-to-toe physical examination and event history are 2 components of a secondary assessment. It is during this stage that details of the child's physical injury are defined and circumstances of the injury are educed.

Comprehensive physical assessment A head-to-toe assessment is an important part of secondary evaluation (**Table 1**).[57] The physical assessment should be thorough and systematic, because multiple injuries may be present and not immediately obvious. To minimize anxiety during the examination, a family member or an adult in whom the child finds comfort should be present to provide support. The nurse should explain steps of the assessment in developmentally appropriate language.

Careful documentation of the physical assessment in the medical record is important in cases in which abuse is suspected. Initial findings provide a baseline for comparison and may be relevant in legal investigations. The comprehensive assessment should be completed at frequent intervals, because new symptoms may emerge throughout the admission to the intensive care unit.

Psychosocial/family assessment Throughout the physical examination, trust and therapeutic rapport can be established with the child and family. It is important to determine the child's emotional and behavioral response to the injury.[17] The psychosocial assessment can also identify child and family sources of stress, coping, and support.[58] The nurse should seek information that identifies both strengths and weaknesses in the child's home environment. Children (who are able to communicate) and families should be asked to describe home routines, living arrangements, and family roles. It is important to establish the habits and activity of those living in the home to identify risk factors consistent with abuse.[58] It is also important to identify the presence of other children in the home who may also be at risk of abusive injury.

The nurse observes the child's behavior, eye contact, and social reaction with staff and family, for important indicators of anxiety, fear, or depression. The child's response to the hospital environment is also important to evaluate. In addition to observing the child's behavior, it is important to observe the family's behavior, interaction, and response to the child and the child's needs. Findings in psychosocial assessment should be carefully documented, in objective nonjudgmental terms. Parents may be able to provide information regarding the child's level of motor, social, and cognitive development, but a comprehensive evaluation should be deferred until the child is medically stable.

Event history: parent The event history is obtained from the accompanying parent or other adult caregiver. There are several factors that affect a parent's level of cooperation in providing information about the injury, including but not limited to:

- Having limited knowledge of the incident
- Having a role in the injury
- Fear in implicating another person in the incident
- Lack of trust with the health care system

The nurse has little control over many factors but can influence the exchange by establishing therapeutic relationship with the family. Introductions, eye contact, information sharing, and active listening are important to this end. The level of trust the nurse is able to garner from the family may affect the level of cooperation and the effort that families put forth in providing an accurate history.

When asking parents to share a description of events, Stirling[59] offers the following 4 pieces of advice:

1. Listen before talking
2. Do not answer your own questions
3. Wait for an answer
4. Retain neutrality

Table 1
Components of head-to-toe physical assessment and significant findings

Area	Components of Assessment	Significant Findings
General	• Vital signs • Pulse oximetry • Height/weight/BMI (>2 y) • General inspection	• Abnormal vital signs for age • Significant underweight/overweight • Cool/diaphoretic skin • Poor hygiene
Head	• Inspect and palpate the head • Inspect the face, ears, neck, and mouth • Inspect the mouth • Level of consciousness, including GCS • Pupils, eye movement, and vision • Evaluate vocalization • Infant fontanels • Muscle tone • Determine strength and symmetry of movement • Observe for posturing • Note pain or tenderness	• Bruising, abrasions, edema, other soft tissue injury • Blood or cerebrospinal fluid in the ears • Missing teeth • Pain • Decreased level of consciousness • Abnormal pupil size or response • High-pitched, weak, or shrill cry; hoarse voice • Full, tense, or bulging fontanels • Flaccid or stiff muscle tone • Asymmetrical movement • Posturing
Chest/Torso	• Inspect anterior and posterior torso • Observe and auscultate respirations • Note respiratory effort • Evaluate skin color • Auscultate cardiac sounds • Palpate peripheral pulses • Evaluate strength and capillary refill time	• Bruising, abrasions, edema, other soft tissue injury • Pain • Increased respiratory rate or effort • Pale skin, mottling, or cyanosis • Abnormal cardiac rhythm • Weak or absent peripheral pulses • Increased capillary refill time
Abdomen	• Inspect the abdomen • Auscultate bowel sounds • Palpate the abdomen • Determine time of last meal • Determine normal bowel pattern and date of last bowel movement • Determine time of last void and urine characteristics	• Abdominal distention • Pain, tenderness, or guarding • Bruising, abrasions, edema, other soft tissue injury • Nausea/vomiting • Frank/occult blood in stool • Frank/occult blood in urine
Perineum	• Inspect the genitalia and buttocks	• Bruising, abrasions, edema, other soft tissue injury • Bleeding
Extremities	• Inspect the extremities • If the child is able, observe gait	• Bruising, abrasions, edema, other soft tissue injury • Pain • Obvious fracture or skeletal misalignment • Limb avoidance or limping

Abbreviations: BMI, body mass index; GCS, Glasgow Coma Scale.
Data from American Heart Association. Pediatric advanced life support: provider manual. American Heart Association; 2011.

Questions and directives should be open-ended to elicit a comprehensive picture of the situation, while not guiding the parent's narrative. The nurse may initiate the exchange with the following:

- Tell me what happened.
- When did you first notice something was wrong?
- Describe the last time you saw the child his or her normal self.

As information is shared, follow-up questions allow for a more complete story to emerge. For example, if the parent reports the child sleeping, the nurse should ask for information on the length and quality of sleep, and inquire about the child's normal sleep routine. If there was a reported fall, the nurse should ask for information about surface height and characteristics and about the child's immediate reaction. The goal is to obtain an accurate and complete history of events that facilitates related diagnosis, treatment, and outcomes.[59] When possible, multiple family members should be questioned separately. Changing details of the account and any facts that are inconsistent with the child's developmental level or degree of physical injury should be noted.

Event history: child Children who are able to communicate should be asked to describe events associated with the injury. When possible, the child should be interviewed separately from the parent.[59] The exchange should proceed in a manner that is sensitive to the individual child, with particular attention to aspects of social and cognitive development. Several factors may prevent a child from open dialogue and disclosure of circumstances surrounding an injury. The nurse can establish trust through active listening, honest information sharing, and communicating respect for both the child and family. When talking with children, Stirling[59] suggests using questions that include simple terms, using proper names instead of pronouns, and addressing only one idea at a time.

American Association of Critical-Care Nurses Standard 2: Diagnosis

The nurse caring for the acutely and critically ill patient analyzes the assessment data in determining diagnosis and care issues.[9]

Needs and deficits are identified in collaboration with the child and family through the nurse's comprehensive assessment. From those needs, a list of priority nursing diagnoses is derived. A list of common nursing diagnoses related to nonaccidental trauma in children is found in **Box 2**. The focus of much nursing care will be related to the physical injury of the child. Emotional and behavioral diagnoses, however, are common for abused children and their families. Acute pain, severe emotional distress, separation from parents, poor social support for the child, use of avoidance or social withdrawal as a coping mechanism, and parental emotional distress, for example, have been associated with both short- and long-term negative outcomes.[17] In recognizing and diagnosing these conditions, the nurse can identify and implement targeted intervention to minimize their effect.

American Association of Critical-Care Nurses Standard 3: Outcomes Identification

The nurse caring for the acutely and critically ill patient identifies outcomes for the patient or the patient's situation.[9]

Expected outcomes of nursing care should be developed in collaboration with the child, participating family, and other providers. Outcomes should be specific for a particular child, be measurable, and include a target date for attainment. Expected outcomes can and should be modified according to a child's changing condition.

Box 2
Common nursing diagnoses associated with nonaccidental trauma

Acute pain

Altered mobility

Anxiety

Caregiver role strain

Deficient knowledge

Delayed growth and development

Excess/deficient fluid volume

Fear

Grieving

Impaired comfort

Impaired parenting

Impaired skin integrity

Impaired social interaction

Impaired tissue integrity

Ineffective airway clearance

Ineffective breathing pattern

Ineffective coping

Ineffective thermoregulation

Moral distress

Parental role conflict

Risk for aspiration

Risk for electrolyte imbalance

Risk for shock

Sleep deprivation

Data from Taylor CM, Ralph SS. Nursing diagnosis reference manual: Sparks and Taylor's. Philadelphia: Lippincott, Williams & Wilkins; 2014.

Based on knowledge of a child's physical condition and available resources, the nurse can help establish realistic and achievable outcome goals.[9]

American Association of Critical-Care Nurses Standard 4: Planning

The nurse caring for the acutely and critically ill patient develops a plan that prescribes interventions to attain outcomes.[9]

In developing the nursing plan of care, attention is given to current standards of best practice and patient and family preference. Interventions based on well-accepted evidence should be implemented. The nursing plan should be developed in collaboration with the child (when developmentally able) and the family. The plan should be individualized to a child's and family's unique needs and resources. The plan should be documented in the child's medical record, so that all nurses provide a consistent plan of care.

Planning interventions to address a child's psychosocial, emotional, and behavioral needs is critically important for children admitted to the hospital for abusive trauma. Hospitalization, in the best of circumstances, can be a stressful experience for children. The nurse should be mindful and purposeful in planning intervention to reduce the effects of this additional burden. Kassam-Adams and colleagues[17] describe 7 key interventions for minimizing the negative psychological sequelae of traumatic injury and hospitalization, including: (1) minimizing traumatic aspects of medical care and procedures, (2) sharing information with the family and child, (3) providing prompt recognition and management of child distress (pain, fear, anxiety), (4) assisting the family to provide emotional support to the child, (5) evaluating family strengths and needs, (6) identifying families that need additional or outside support, and (7) assisting children to identify and practice effective coping mechanisms. These interventions are components of an approach called trauma-informed pediatric care, in which providers are consciously aware of the risk of adverse psychological outcomes for children who have experienced a traumatic event.[17]

An interdisciplinary care team, which includes a child's family, is important for any child with complex needs.[33] The nurse should ensure that a wide variety of specialties are involved in the child's care, by initiating consultation and recommending other members to the team as needs arise. Social workers should be a primary member of the interdisciplinary team, because they play an important role in coordinating care for children who have been abused.[60] Social workers often serve as a liaison between the health care system and legal systems of child protection, by ensuring that relevant communication is shared.[60] Social workers provide advocacy for the injured child throughout the hospital stay and work with legal and social agencies to identify a safe home environment for discharge. In addition to social workers, a host of other specialists should be considered in developing a holistic plan of care for children, based on the child's and family's individual needs (**Box 3**).[16]

Box 3
Members of the interdisciplinary team

- Family
- Nurses
- Physicians/surgeons
- Social workers
- Child life specialists
- Chaplains/spiritual support
- Pharmacists
- Dieticians
- Case managers
- Pain specialists
- Trauma specialists
- Palliative care specialists
- Respiratory therapists
- Occupational, speech, and physical therapists

Family care conferences can be particularly helpful in engaging families and helping families set goals and make decisions about care. Decision making may also be complicated by pending legal cases involving the parents, so a multidisciplinary team is required.[61] There is little in the literature that describes the role of care conferences with respect to cases of abusive trauma. However, their role in facilitating communication in the intensive care unit, particularly around issues of end-of-life decisions is recognized.[61,62]

American Association of Critical-Care Nurses Standard 5: Implementation

The nurse caring for the acutely and critically ill patient implements the plan, coordinates care delivery, and employs strategies to promote health and a safe environment.[9]

Once the plan has been derived, the nurse works with other members of the health care team to implement it. Caring for parents and families who may have been involved in causing the child's injury creates an appreciable paradox for the nurse. Nurses describe conflict in caring for the child-family unit, while maintaining the role of child advocate.[5] Despite the inner conflict it causes the nurse, the family continues to hold a central role in the child's life.[63] The family may be fraught with dysfunction, but it is what the child knows, and children often find comfort in what is known. Principles of family-centered care arise from this core belief and as a result can be applied even in cases of abusive trauma.[63]

The nurse's role in the intensive care unit is to ensure the child's safe interaction with the family. Legally mandated visitor restrictions must be observed. The nurse should carefully observe and objectively document all family visits and interaction, including their duration, activity, and the child's response. Physical presence of a parent does not ensure that parental role is filled for the child. As Livesley[64] states, "parental residence is no guarantee of parental presence, and parental presence is no guarantee of emotional availability."

For a child who is unaccompanied in the hospital, by virtue of parental neglect or legal mandate, nurses fill the caregiver void.[64] Filling the role of missing parent can create a situation in which roles can become blurred. Nurses in this situation report a need to clearly distinguish and differentiate their role as nurse from that of parent.[64]

American Association of Critical-Care Nurses Standard 6: Evaluation

The nurse caring for the acutely and critically ill patient evaluates progress toward attaining outcomes.[9]

Evaluation of progress toward outcomes should be an iterative process and continue throughout the length of stay in the pediatric intensive care unit. Effectiveness of selected nursing interventions should be evaluated. As progress and outcomes are evaluated or new concerns arise, diagnoses, expected outcomes, plans, and interventions should be modified to address the changing conditions.

SUMMARY

Child abuse is an odious societal reality, and pediatric nurses have an important part to play. Each year thousands of children are hospitalized for traumatic injuries associated with physical abuse. Nurses in the pediatric intensive care unit must be knowledgeable and skilled in caring for the physical, psychological, emotional, social, and developmental needs of physically abused children and their families. Through adherence to the broad standards outlined by the AACN, nurses in an intensive care setting can provide nursing care that maximizes health outcomes and minimizes the negative consequence of abuse for children and their families.

REFERENCES

1. U. S. Department of Health and Human Services, Administration for Children and Families, Administration on Children, Youth and Families, Children's Bureau. (2013). Child maltreatment 2012. Available at: http://www.acf.hhs.gov/sites/default/files/cb/cm2012.pdf. Accessed November 1, 2015.
2. Farst K, Ambadwar PB, King AJ, et al. Trends in hospitalization rates and severity of injuries from abuse in young children, 1997-2009. Pediatrics 2013;131:e1796–802.
3. Leventhal JM, Martin KD, Gaither JR. Using US data to estimate the incidence of serious physical abuse in children. Pediatrics 2012;129:458–64.
4. DeMattei R, Sherry J, Rogers J, et al. What future health care providers will need to know about child abuse and neglect. Health Care Manag 2009;28:320–7.
5. Tingberg B, Bredlov B, Ygge B. Nurses' experience in clinical encounters with children experiencing abuse and their parents. J Clin Nurs 2008;17:2718–24.
6. Schwartz KA, Preer G, McKeag H, et al. Child maltreatment: a review of key literature in 2013. Curr Opin Pediatr 2014;26:396–404.
7. Lyden C. Caring for the victim of child abuse in the pediatric intensive care unit. Dimens Crit Care Nurs 2009;28:61–6.
8. Zenel J, Goldstein B. Child abuse in the pediatric intensive care unit. Crit Care Med 2002;30:S515–23.
9. American Association of Critical Care Nurses. AACN scope and standards for acute and critical care nursing practice. Aliso Viejo (CA): American Association of Critical Care Nurses; 2008.
10. Douglas EM, Mohn BL. Fatal and non-fatal child maltreatment in the US: an analysis of child, caregiver, and service utilization with the National Child Abuse and Neglect Data Set. Child Abuse Negl 2014;38:42–51.
11. Jones L, Bellis MA, Wood S, et al. Prevalence and risk of violence against children with disabilities: a systematic review and meta-analysis of observational studies. Lancet 2012;380:899–907.
12. Anderson T, DeCarlo A, Voisin D, et al. Trauma and violence in childhood: a U.S. perspective. Psychiatr Times 2003;20:91.
13. Dube SR, Felitti VJ, Dong M, et al. The impact of adverse childhood experiences on health problems: evidence from four birth cohorts dating back to 1900. Prev Med 2003;37:268–77.
14. Perry BD. The neurodevelopmental impact of violence in childhood. In: Schetky D, Benedek EP, editors. Textbook of Child and Adolescent Forensic Psychiatry. Washington, DC: American Psychiatric Press, Inc.; 2001. p. 221–38.
15. Draper B, Pfaff J, Pirkis J, et al. Long-term effects of childhood abuse on the quality of life and health of older people: results from the depression and early prevention of suicide in general practice project. J Am Geriatr Soc 2008;56:262–71.
16. Mulvihill D. Nursing care of children after a traumatic accident. Issues Compr Pediatr Nurs 2007;30:15–28.
17. Kassam-Adams N, Rzucidlo S, Campbell M, et al. Nurses' views and current practice of trauma-informed pediatric nursing care. J Pediatr Nurs 2014;23:51–9.
18. Felitti VJ, Anda RF, Nordenberg D, et al. Relationship of childhood abuse and household dysfunction to many of the leading causes of death in adults. The adverse childhood experiences (ACE) study. Am J Prev Med 1998;14:245–58.

19. Gabbay V, Oatis MD, Silva RR, et al. Epidemiological aspects of PTSD in children and adolescents. In: Silva Raul R, editor. Posttraumatic stress disorder in children and adolescents: handbook. New York: Norton; 2004. p. 1–17.
20. Scott M, Palmer S, editors. Trauma and posttraumatic stress disorder. New York: Cassell; 2000.
21. Jacobi G, Dettmeyer R, Banaschak S, et al. Child abuse and neglect: diagnosis and management. Dtsch Arztebl Int 2010;107:231–40.
22. Krysinska K, Lester D, Martin G. Suicidal behavior after a traumatic event. J Trauma Nurs 2009;16(2):103–10.
23. American Psychological Association. Children and trauma: APA presidential task force on posttraumatic stress disorder and trauma in children & adolescents. 2009. Available at: http://www.apa.org/pi/families/resources/children-trauma.pdf. Accessed November 1, 2015.
24. Deans KJ, Thackeray J, Groner JI, et al. Risk factors for recurrent injuries in victims of suspected non-accidental trauma: a retrospective cohort study. BMC Pediatr 2014;14:217.
25. Child Welfare Information Gateway. Mandatory reporters of child abuse and neglect. 2014. Available at: https://www.childwelfare.gov/systemwide/laws_policies/statutes/manda.pdf. Accessed November 1, 2015.
26. Parks SE, Annest JL, Hill HA, et al. Pediatric abusive head trauma: recommended definitions for public health surveillance and research. Atlanta (GA): Centers for Disease Control and Prevention; 2012.
27. Kemp AM, Jaspan T, Griffiths J, et al. Neuroimaging: what neuroradiological features distinguish abusive from non-abusive head trauma? A systematic review. Arch Dis Child 2011;96:1103–12.
28. Xiang J, Shi J, Wheeler KK, et al. Paediatric patients with abusive head trauma treated in US emergency departments, 2006-2009. Brain Inj 2013;27:1555–61.
29. Gordy C, Kuns B. Pediatric abusive head trauma. Nurs Clin North Am 2013;48:193–201.
30. Selassie AW, Borg K, Busch C, et al. Abusive head trauma in young children. J Trauma Nurs 2014;29:72–82.
31. Acker SN, Partrick DA, Ross JT, et al. Head injury and unclear mechanism of injury: Initial hematocrit less than 30 is predictive of abusive head trauma in young children. J Pediatr Surg 2014;49:338–40.
32. Shein SL, Bell MJ, Kochanek PM, et al. Risk factors for mortality in children with abusive head trauma. J Pediatr 2012;161:716–22.
33. Christian CW, Block R, The American Academy of Pediatrics Committee on Child Abuse and Neglect. Abusive head trauma in infants and children. Pediatrics 2009;123:1409–11.
34. Barlow K, Thompson E, Johnson D, et al. The neurological outcome of non-accidental head injury. Pediatr Rehabil 2004;7:195–203.
35. Barlow K, Thompson E, Johnson D, et al. Late neurologic and cognitive sequelae of inflicted traumatic brain injury in infancy. Pediatrics 2005;116:e174–85.
36. Hymel KP, Armijo-Garcia V, Foster R, et al. Validation of a clinical prediction rule for pediatric abusive head trauma. Pediatrics 2014;134:e1537–44.
37. Narang S, Clarke J. Abusive head trauma: past, present, and future. J Child Neurol 2014;29:1747–56.
38. Piteau SJ, Ward MG, Barrowman NJ, et al. Clinical and radiographic characteristics associated with abusive and nonabusive head trauma: a systematic review. Pediatrics 2012;130:315–23.

39. Richardson NC, Rappaport DI. Pediatric head trauma: abuse of not? Hosp Pediatr 2012;2:247–8.
40. Roach JP, Acker SN, Bensard DD, et al. Head injury pattern in children can help differentiate accidental from non-accidental trauma. Pediatr Surg Int 2014;30: 1103–6.
41. Lane WG, Lotwin I, Dubowitz H, et al. Outcomes for children hospitalized with abusive versus noninflicted abdominal trauma. Pediatrics 2011;127: e1400–5.
42. Pariset JM, Feldman KW, Paris C. The pace of signs and symptoms of blunt abdominal trauma to children. Clin Pediatr 2010;49:24–8.
43. Lane WG, Dubowitz H, Langenberg P, et al. Epidemiology of abusive abdominal trauma hospitalizations in United States children. Child Abuse Negl 2012;36: 142–8.
44. Terreros A, Zimmerman S. Duodenal hematoma from a fall down the stairs. J Trauma Nurs 2009;16:166–8.
45. Maguire SA, Upadhyaya M, Evans A, et al. A systematic review of abusive visceral injuries in childhood: their range and recognition. Child Abuse Negl 2013;37:430–45.
46. Trokel M, Discala C, Terrin NC, et al. Patient and injury characteristics in abusive abdominal injuries. Pediatr Emerg Care 2006;22:700–4.
47. Asilioglu N, Paksu MS, Sungur M, et al. Intracardiac thrombus case caused by blunt trauma due to child abuse. Pediatr Emerg Care 2012;28:566–7.
48. Lane WG, Dubowitz H, Langenberg P. Screening for occult abdominal trauma in children with suspected physical abuse. Pediatrics 2009;124:1595–602.
49. Flaherty EG, Perez-Rossello JM, Levine MA, et al. Evaluating children with fractures for child physical abuse. Pediatrics 2014;133:e477–89.
50. Jayakumar P, Barry M, Ramachandran M. Orthopaedic aspects of paediatric non accidental injury. J Bone Joint Surg Br 2010;92:189–95.
51. Leventhal JM, Martin KD, Asnes AG. Incidence of fractures attributable to abuse in young hospitalized children: results from a united states database. Pediatrics 2008;122:599–604.
52. Kemp AM, Dunstan F, Harrison S, et al. Patterns of skeletal fractures in child abuse: systematic review. BMJ 2008;337:1518.
53. Wood JN, Fakeye O, Mondestin V, et al. Prevalence of abuse among young children with femur fractures: a systematic review. BMC Pediatr 2014;14:169.
54. Clarke NM, Shelton FR, Taylor CC, et al. The incidence of fractures in children under the age of 24 months – in relation to non-accidental injury. Injury 2012; 43:762–5.
55. Ravichandiran N, Schuh S, Bejuk M, et al. Delayed identification of pediatric abuse-related fractures. Pediatrics 2010;125:60–6.
56. American Heart Association. Pediatric advanced life support: provider manual. Dallas (TX): American Heart Association; 2011.
57. Pasek TA, Etzel KA. Multiple trauma. In: Slota MC, editor. Core curriculum for pediatric critical care nursing. St Louis (MO): Elsevier; 2006. p. 638–87.
58. Pierce MC, Kaczor K, Thompson R. Bringing back the social history. Pediatr Clin North Am 2014;61:889–905.
59. Stirling J. The conversation: interacting with parents when child abuse is suspected. Pediatr Clin North Am 2014;61:979–95.
60. Connolly S. Everyone's business: developing an integrated model of care to respond to child abuse in a pediatric hospital setting. Soc Work Health Care 2012;51:36–52.

61. Ellingson CC, Livingston JS, Fanaroff JM. End-of-life decisions in abusive head trauma. Pediatrics 2012;129:541–7.
62. Michelson KN, Emanuel L, Carter A, et al. Pediatric intensive care unit family conference: one mode of communication for discussing end-of-life care decisions. Pediatr Crit Care Med 2011;12:e336–43.
63. Barton SJ. Family-centered care when abuse or neglect is suspected. J Spec Pediatr Nurs 2000;5:96–9.
64. Livesley J. Telling tales: a qualitative exploration of how children's nurses interpret work with unaccompanied hospitalized children. J Clin Nurs 2005;14:43–50.

Trauma in the Geriatric Population

Cathy A. Maxwell, PhD, RN

KEYWORDS

- Geriatric trauma • Injured older adults • Epidemiology
- Evidence-based management • Frailty • Advanced care planning • Injury prevention

KEY POINTS

- Geriatric trauma is a looming public health crisis with implications for clinicians, health care administrators, policymakers, and society at large.
- Characteristics and risk factors related to geriatric trauma differ significantly from younger adults.
- Patient management of injured older adults should be regarded from a continuum of care perspective, including triage, transport, initial assessment, inpatient care, and hospital discharge.
- An understanding of frailty, advanced care planning, and end-of-life care are important considerations because injury is often a tipping point leading to functional decline and poor outcomes.
- Injury prevention efforts in older adults focus on fall prevention and driver safety programs.

INTRODUCTION

The prevalence of geriatric trauma is increasing in the United States as Baby Boomers reach age 65. Soon, the percentage of adults aged 65 and older will climb from 13.7% (2013) to 21% (2040),[1] with significant societal implications. A review of geriatric trauma as a distinct entity under the broader umbrella of traumatic injury is timely and warranted. Injury in later life and the resulting sequelae call for an understanding of characteristics and risk factors unique to older adults, as well as for awareness of evidence-based guidelines for risk assessment, goal-directed care, and injury prevention.

EPIDEMIOLOGY OF GERIATRIC TRAUMA

Incidence and distribution of traumatic injury in older adults differ from younger adults **(Table 1)**. Older adults (aged ≥65) are hospitalized for injury more often than younger adults despite lower injury severity.[2] Of injured younger adults, 70% are discharged

The author has no conflicts of interest.
Vanderbilt University School of Nursing, 461 21st Avenue South – GH 420, Nashville, TN 37240, USA
E-mail address: cathy.maxwell@vanderbilt.edu

Table 1
Hospitalizations in the United States with primary injury diagnoses (2012)

2012 National Statistics Healthcare Cost and Utilization Project (HCUPnet)[a]	n (%)	Inpatient Length of Stay (d), Mean	Inpatient Charges (Mean)	Inpatient Mortality (%), Mean	Percentage of Patients Discharged Home
Adults (aged 18–64)	647,510 (48)	5.1	$65,764	1.7	70.5
Adults (aged ≥65)	711,120 (52)	5.1	$49,849	3.2	18.0
Total (all adults)	1,358,630 (100)	5.1	$57,807	2.5	44.3

[a] All adults admitted to US hospitals with a primary injury diagnosis (ICD9 codes: 800.0–959.9).
From Agency for Healthcare Research and Quality (AHRQ). Healthcare Cost and Utilization Project (HCUPnet). 2012. Available at: http://hcupnet.ahrq.gov. Accessed October 23, 2014.

home, compared with only 18% of older injured adults.[2] Hospital charges for care of younger adults are higher (reflecting higher injury severity) than older adults. Falls account for approximately 65% of older adult injuries, whereas motor vehicle traumas are predominant in younger individuals.[3] Likewise, falls are the leading cause of unintentional injury deaths in older adults, followed by motor vehicle events (**Fig. 1**).[4]

Although the prevalence and incidence of elder abuse are relatively small and difficult to estimate, the most recent study, *The National Elder Mistreatment Study* (conducted in 2008) reported overall prevalence of elder physical mistreatment to be 1.6% of adults aged 60 and older.[5] Types of physical mistreatment included hitting (1.2%), restraining (0.4%), and other injury (0.7%). The prevalence of other forms of mistreatment included emotional mistreatment (4.6%), sexual mistreatment (0.6%), potential neglect (5.1%), and financial mistreatment (5.2%).[5]

Table 2 summarizes types of primary injuries incurred by older adults admitted to US hospitals in 2012.[2] Lower extremity fractures (including hip fractures) are the most common injuries (47%), followed by injuries to the neck and trunk (18%), including rib fractures and vertebral fractures. Patients with head injuries have the longest hospital stay, followed by those with spinal cord injuries and internal injuries

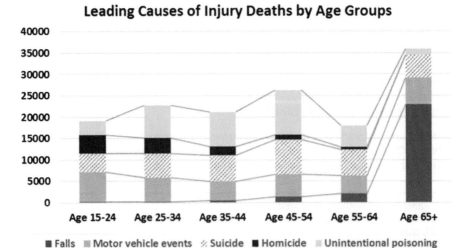

Leading Causes of Injury Deaths by Age Groups

■ Falls   ■ Motor vehicle events   ▨ Suicide   ■ Homicide   ▨ Unintentional poisoning

Fig. 1. Leading causes of unintentional injury deaths by age groups (2011). (*From* Centers for Disease Control and Prevention. Injury prevention and control: data and statistics (WISQAR). Available at: http://www.cdc.gov/injury/wisqars/. Accessed September 15, 2014.)

Table 2
Primary injuries and patient outcomes related to geriatric trauma

2012 National Statistics Healthcare Cost and Utilization Project (HCUPnet)[a] (Primary Injury)	n (%)	Inpatient Length of Stay (d), Mean	Inpatient Charges (Mean)	Inpatient Mortality (%), Mean	Percentage of Patients Discharged Home (%)
Lower extremity fractures	332,545 (47)	5.4	$54,204	2.2	6
Neck and trunk fractures	129,810 (18)	5.0	$42,305	2.2	19
Intracranial injuries	83,185 (12)	5.3	$54,196	9.3	30
Upper extremity fractures	59,140 (8)	3.9	$42,714	0.6	30
Skull fractures	18,440 (3)	5.8	$60,326	10.7	33
Internal injuries of the thorax/abdomen/pelvis	17,170 (2)	6.7	$63,560	6.5	39
Contusions	16,095 (2)	4.1	$27,297	0.8	31
Sprains and strains	10,770 (1)	3.3	$28,958	0.4	40
Injuries to nerves and spinal cord	1755 (<1)	8.4	$99,769	6.6	24
Superficial injuries	1165 (<1)	3.4	$20,901	0.9	50
Other[b]	41,045 (6)	—	—	—	—
Total	711,120 (100)	5.1	$48,849	3.2	18

Statistics are based on primary ICD9 codes reported in medical records to state databases.
[a] Patients (aged ≥65) admitted to US hospitals with a primary injury diagnosis (ICD9 codes: 800.0–959.9).
[b] Other: Open wounds (2%), injury to blood vessels (<1%), late effects of injuries (<1%), burns (<1%), dislocations (<1%), crushing injuries (<1%), foreign bodies (<1%), unspecified injuries (<1%).
From Agency for Healthcare Research and Quality (AHRQ). Healthcare Cost and Utilization Project (HCUPnet). 2012. Available at: http://hcupnet.ahrq.gov. Accessed October 23, 2014.

to the thorax, abdomen, and pelvis. Mean inpatient charges range from $20,901 (superficial injuries) to $99,769 (injuries to nerves and spinal cord). Inpatient mortality is highest for skull fractures (10.7%) and intracranial injuries (9.3%). Discharges to home settings are less than 50% for every injury category, with only 6% of older adults with lower extremity fractures discharged home. These statistics highlight the role of postacute care after geriatric trauma, as well as the need to optimize transitions of care across facilities to prevent costly readmissions.

RESOURCES FOR GERIATRIC TRAUMA CARE

Aging involves physiologic changes and progressive decline in organ systems. Numerous resources focus on physiologic characteristics unique to older adults. This review focuses on aspects of care that are particularly applicable to geriatric trauma by incorporating resources developed by leaders within the trauma care community and reporting on factors of greatest relevance. Recently published, *Geriatric Trauma and Critical Care*, edited by Yelon and Luchette,[6] provides an overview of management of older adults with surgical pathology, with an emphasis on traumatic injury (**Fig. 2**). Thirty-two chapters address 4 categories:

1. Impact of aging on health;
2. Surgical emergencies in the elderly;
3. Traumatic injury in the elderly; and
4. Critical care management of the elderly.

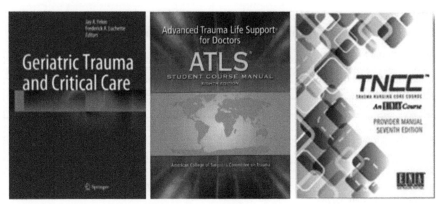

Fig. 2. Resources for geriatric trauma management.

Authored by leaders in trauma care, the book provides a definitive resource for multiple disciplines in assessment and inpatient management of older adults. Particular attention is given to ethical issues related to aging.

The American College of Surgeons (ACS) first recognized trauma care as a distinct entity in the 1980s. Now in its 6th edition, *Resources for Optimal Care of the Injured Patient*[7] was first published in 1990 and recognized geriatric trauma as a category of trauma care warranting special attention. Developed by the ACS, the Advanced Trauma Life Support course[8] for physicians includes a module on geriatric trauma, as does the Emergency Nurses Association–sponsored Trauma Nurse Core Course.[9] Both courses review pertinent physiologic characteristics unique to older adults, as well as guidelines for care (see **Fig. 2**).

The Eastern Association for the Surgery of Trauma (EAST) develops and updates practice management guidelines for categories of trauma surgery, including geriatric trauma.[10,11] Guidelines are based on systematic reviews of literature, classified according to levels of evidence (class I, randomized controlled trials; class II, prospective and retrospective analyses from clearly reliable data; class III, studies from retrospective data, case reviews, and expert opinion).[12] The most recent EAST guidelines for geriatric trauma (2012) advocate for aggressive triage of older trauma patients to trauma centers that have attained excellence in the care of injured patients. The guidelines also promote early assessment of coagulation profiles to correct coagulopathies in patients who take anticoagulants. Last, EAST guidelines advocate for early assessment of base deficit in older patients as a marker of severe injury.

The ACS Trauma Quality Improvement Program also publishes Geriatric Trauma Management Guidelines (2013) aimed at improving trauma care among injured older adults.[13] Based on best available evidence, these guidelines address the continuum of care for the hospitalized injured older adult.

Consistent with a continuum of care approach, the following sections address evidence-based management of geriatric trauma, including triage and transport, trauma team activation and initial assessment, inpatient care, frailty, pain management, cognitive impairment, nutrition, advanced care planning, and discharge.

TRIAGE AND TRANSPORT

Although risk of death after injury increases after age 55,[14] a disproportionate percentage of injured older adults are transported to nontrauma centers compared with younger adults.[15–17] Undertriage of older patients to nontrauma centers is associated with an increased risk of mortality.[18] Patients in oldest age groups treated at non-trauma centers with severe injuries, including head injuries, have higher inpatient mortality than those treated at verified trauma centers.[16,19] In light of this evidence, the ACS Committee on Trauma recommends consideration of transport to trauma centers for injured patients aged 55 or older, particularly those with injuries in more than 1 body region, as well as those with more severe injuries.[7]

TRAUMA TEAM ACTIVATION AND INITIAL ASSESSMENT

Assessment of the geriatric trauma patient entails attention to not only injury-specific interventions, but also geriatric-specific considerations. Trauma teams consist of physicians, nurses, and other health care providers, led by a team captain who ensures rapid assessment and interventional care upon arrival to an emergency department. Trauma team activation ensures a thorough and systematic assessment of injured patients that includes primary, secondary, and tertiary evaluations. Consideration of an age threshold for trauma team activation in older patients (ie, patients ages ≥ 70 years) may mitigate late recognition of injuries that might otherwise be missed.[20] The initial evaluation of injured older adults should include attention to home medications and consideration of conditions unique to older adults. Proactive assessment for and recognition of other nontraumatic conditions unique to older adults (geriatric syndromes, common comorbidities) may preempt additional complications during hospitalization. Fallon and colleagues[21] demonstrated improved outcomes for geriatric trauma patients who were assessed and followed by a geriatrician, including recognition and management of delirium, pain management, advanced care planning, and medication management.

A significant percentage of older adults take anticoagulants and antiplatelet agents to lower the risk of stroke; preinjury use of these medications increases risk of bleeding complications.[22–24] Evaluation of anticoagulant use should occur during initial patient assessment, along with pertinent laboratory tests (prothrombin time, partial thromboplastin time, international normalized ratio). Geriatric trauma guidelines recommend protocols that ensure rapid head CT and early correction of elevated international normalized ratios through use of fresh frozen plasma and vitamin K.[12,13] Correction of international normalized ratio values to less than 1.6 is recommended. The ACS notes that this field of research is rapidly changing and that newer guidelines may emerge as our understanding of outcomes related to coagulopathies increases.[13]

Other medications can influence patient assessment and management, including β-blockers and angiotensin-converting enzyme inhibitors. β-Blockers are noted to blunt the stress response to shock and can mask underlying hypoperfusion.[25] Angiotensin-converting enzyme inhibitors should be continued during hospitalization; however, the dose should be adjusted according to renal function.[13] For laboratory assessment of the geriatric trauma patient, clinicians should consider a lactic acid or blood gas (for base deficit), coagulation profile, blood urea nitrogen, creatinine, blood alcohol level, urine toxicology screen, and serum electrolytes. Imaging studies should include all CT scans to rule out potential or suspected injuries.[13]

INPATIENT CARE FOR GERIATRIC TRAUMA

Assessment for geriatric-specific conditions and potential complications is paramount during hospitalization of injured older adults. Min and colleagues[26] identified mortality-associated complications in injured older adults, including wound infections, urinary tract infections, pneumonia, pressure ulcers, and deep vein thrombosis. Early comprehensive geriatric assessment and/or consultation by a geriatrician provides opportunity for recognition of geriatric syndromes and optimal management of age-related conditions. Geriatric syndromes are defined as conditions that do not fit into common disease categories, yet occur in older adults and have the potential to significantly affect quality of life (**Box 1**).

FRAILTY

Geriatric trauma patients at greatest risk for complications and poor outcomes are those deemed frail.[27,28] Frailty is a syndrome of vulnerability affecting up to 65% of hospitalized, injured older adults.[29] Frailty is defined as a condition of vulnerability characterized by poor resolution of homeostasis after a stressor event that is a consequence of cumulative decline in many physiologic systems over a lifetime.[30] Frail older adults have reached a stage in which an external stressor of injury is often a tipping point that initiates subsequent decline that can lead to death. Thus, frailty assessment should be an early priority of inpatient care. Assessment for frailty upon hospital admission provides pertinent information for individualized, goal-directed care. Experts in frailty research maintain that physical frailty is a manageable condition that is reversible through targeted interventions (ie, exercise, caloric and protein support, vitamin D, reduction in polypharmacy).[30]

Recommendations from a 2012 consensus conference on frailty include the need for all persons older than age 70 to be screened for frailty.[31] Several brief screening instruments for detection of frailty are available to clinicians (**Box 2**). The feasibility of screening injured older adults for preinjury frailty has been established; however, the presence of surrogate respondents is a noted necessity.[29,32] Screening instruments are designed to trigger further assessment and should not be used for diagnostic purposes because most address single domains or factors related to frailty (eg, physical activity, strength, cognition). A thorough, multidimensional assessment by a clinician with geriatric expertise is recommended.

PAIN MANAGEMENT

Pain control after traumatic injury is crucial in the elderly. Considerations related to pain management in older adults include (1) use of appropriate analgesics, (2) early use of nonnarcotic pain medications, (3) epidural analgesia for patients with multiple rib fractures, and (4) avoidance of benzodiazepines. The Beers criteria for potentially

---

Box 1
Common geriatric syndromes

- Falls
- Urinary incontinence
- Delirium
- Pressure ulcers
- Urinary tract infections
- Eating and/or feeding problems
- Sleep problems
- Polypharmacy
- Pain
- Sarcopenia and frailty

Box 2
Brief screening instruments for identification of frailty in older adults

- Vulnerable Elders Survey[33]
- Barthel Index[34]
- Life Space Assessment[35]
- Katz Activities of Daily Living[36]
- Frailty Index[37]
- Gérontopôle Frailty Screening Tool[38]
- The simple FRAIL Questionnaire Screening Tool[39]
- Cardiovascular Health Study Frailty Screening Scale[40]

Data from Refs.[33–40]

---

inappropriate medication use in older adults provides guidance for use of defined categories of drugs.[41] Meperidine should not be used because it can cause neurotoxicity, and safer choices are available. Other oral nonsteroidal antiinflammatory drugs should be used with caution because they can increase the risk of gastrointestinal bleeding. Muscle relaxants are not recommended for older adults because they have anticholinergic effects and can cause oversedation. Acceptable nonnarcotic analgesics include dipyrone, acetaminophen, and tramadol. Oxycodone may be used for severe pain, but should not be used as a first-choice analgesic. Epidural catheters are preferred for pain control in older patients with multiple rib fractures because they avoid side effects of oral and intravenous narcotics and are associated with reduced mortality in some studies.[42] Use of benzodiazepines in older adults can increase risk of cognitive impairment (ie, delirium) that can lead to falls, resulting in further injury.

COGNITIVE IMPAIRMENT

Cognitive impairments in injured older adults prevent optimal communication of patient wishes regarding treatment and advanced care planning. Dementia is present in one-third of hospitalized older adults,[43] and delirium is reported in up to 37% of injured patients.[32] Family caregivers play a primary role when patients are unable to make informed decisions regarding treatment choices. Clinicians should seek the most appropriate surrogate who can truly represent patient preferences. Palliative care services are helpful in guiding family caregivers through complex decisions that entail discussions about postinjury risks, potential complications, functional decline, mortality, advanced directives, comfort measures, and end-of-life care.

Delirium, or acute confusion with inattention, occurs in up to 30% of hospitalized older adults,[44] and is greatest in the oldest age groups.[45] Delirium places older patients at risk for adverse events, prolonged hospitalization, and increased mortality. Risk factors for delirium include pain, infection, sedative use, surgery, electrolyte disturbances, hypoxic events, and nutritional deficiencies. Many screening instruments are available to clinicians for detection of delirium. The Confusion Assessment Method (CAM)[46] and CAM-ICU[47] are the most widely used instruments for screening and diagnosis of delirium. Prevention of delirium is best accomplished through recognition of patients at risk. Interventions for prevention and treatment include multiple components aimed at normalizing a patient's environment, early mobilization, and correction of predisposing factors.

NUTRITION

Malnutrition and weight loss among hospitalized older adults occur in up to 20% of patients.[48] Older trauma patients, particularly those who are frail, are often malnourished at the time of injury, placing them at greater risk for further decline. Older patients often have diminished appetite, presenting an additional challenge during hospitalization. Screening for malnutrition at hospital admission entails questions about appetite, digestive problems, weight loss, and swallowing difficulties. Early nutritional assessments are aimed at meeting energy (caloric and protein) requirements of 120% to 140% of predicted basal energy expenditure.[49] Such an approach has been shown to improve patient outcomes.[49,50]

ADVANCED CARE PLANNING

The changing demographics of geriatric trauma have placed increased focus on quality of life and endpoints of care. Geriatric trauma patients and their families are often faced with difficult decisions related to life-sustaining measures and end-of-life care. Facing these decisions in conjunction with unexpected trauma creates sensitive and challenging scenarios. Although trauma care providers have expertise in injury management, few resources specific to geriatric trauma are available to facilitate family discussions regarding advanced care planning and palliative care. Advanced care planning involves an understanding that these difficult decisions are best made ahead of time. Consideration of specific decisions, including cardiopulmonary resuscitation, ventilator use, artificial nutrition and hydration, and comfort care ensure that patient preferences are honored. Leaders within the trauma care community advocate for development of geriatric trauma prediction models to encourage and facilitate these discussions.[12,51]

The National Institute on Aging suggests the use of potential scenarios by health care providers to facilitate understanding of the need for advanced care planning. For example, a provider might describe a specific scenario that describes a poor health state with the potential for poor outcomes. Then, the provider would ask the patient or caregiver to imagine themselves in the scenario and to choose the option that would best represent their wishes. **Box 3** provides an example of a geriatric trauma scenario that might be used to discuss advanced care planning. Treatment options may range from full life support treatments to no life support. Using such scenarios, Sudore and colleagues[52] conducted a study with more than 200 chronically ill English- and Spanish-speaking older adults and reported more uncertainty among Latinos and Asians compared with Whites, and advocated for culturally sensitive, literacy appropriate tools to address decisional uncertainty. Future work is needed to determine optimal approaches for culturally based, patient-centered care.

DISCHARGE FROM ACUTE CARE

A significant percentage (70%–80%)[2,32] of injured older adults is transferred to other facilities after initial hospitalization, including rehabilitation facilities, skilled nursing facilities, assisted living, long-term acute care, and inpatient hospice care. Attention to postacute care after hospitalization is warranted particularly in injured older adults. Optimizing transitions of care among facilities improves overall management and prevents inadvertent omissions that can lead to readmissions. Transitions of care are changes in level, location, or providers of care as patients are transferred from 1 facility or unit to another. Medicare patients' rehospitalizations within 30 days of discharge are as high as 20%.[53] Patient readmissions from skilled nursing facilities are as high as 25%.[54] Coordination of care between facilities is often lacking because providers

> **Box 3**
> **Geriatric trauma advanced care planning scenario**
>
> I am going to describe a scenario that occurs here on our trauma unit, and I want you to imagine what it would be like if you (or your loved one) were in this same situation. Imagine the doctor telling you that the severity of your chest and extremity injuries, along with your other conditions (congestive heart failure) before the injury, was such that you needed to be placed on a breathing machine (ventilator) and that it would be difficult to wean you off the machine once you were on it. Suppose the doctor told you that your prognosis was poor and that you may die within the next 6 months. You are faced with deciding what to do.
>
> Your doctor thinks that life-sustaining measures are not likely to help you live longer and that they may cause you to experience additional pain or other discomfort. Life-sustaining measures include shocks to the heart, pressing on the chest (CPR), a tube placed in the lungs to connect to a breathing machine, a tube placed in the nose to your stomach to help with feeding.
>
> Based on my description, would you still want to receive all life-sustaining measures? Would you want only some measures? Would you prefer that no life-sustaining measures be done and that we focus on your wishes for comfort in the setting of your choice?
>
> *Adapted from* Sudore RL, Schillinger D, Knight SJ, et al. Uncertainty about advance care planning treatment preferences among diverse older adults. J Health Commun 2010;15(S2):161.

are accustomed to working in single venues or "silos" and do not feel responsible for what happens to patients once they leave their site.[55] Li and colleagues[56] identified 5 common themes that contribute to poor coordination of care (**Box 4**).

Several transitions of care models are described within the literature to guide and improve transitions of care among settings (**Box 5**). From a systematic review of literature, Hansen and colleagues[57] reported interventions that reduce 30-day rehospitalizations in 3 categories: predischarge, postdischarge, and bridging interventions. **Box 6** lists strategies to reduce hospital readmissions.

INJURY PREVENTION

Injury prevention efforts related to geriatric trauma center around fall prevention and driver safety programs. On a personal level, falls threaten independence, lead to functional decline, and shorten life expectancy. At a societal level, falls generate economic costs that will reach more than $54 billion dollars by 2020.[67] The National Council on Aging (NCOA) serves as the primary coordinating body for fall prevention efforts.[68] NCOA advances the implementation and dissemination of evidence-based fall prevention programs to reduce the incidence of falls. Factors associated with falls include balance and

> **Box 4**
> **Themes that contribute to poor coordination of care across settings**
>
> - Poor provider communication
> - Ineffective patient and caregiver education
> - No follow-up with primary care providers
> - Failure to address chronic conditions
> - Lack of community support
>
> *Data from* Li J, Young R, Williams MV. Optimizing transitions of care to reduce rehospitalizations. Cleve Clin J Med 2014;81(5):313–4.

Box 5
National models of best practices for transitions of care

- Project BOOST: Better Outcomes by Optimizing Safe Transitions[58]
- Project RED: Re-Engineered Discharge[59]
- STAAR: State Action on Avoidable Re-hospitalizations[60]
- The Care Transitions Program[61]
- Transitional Care Model[62]
- The Bridge Model[63]
- Guided Care[64]
- GRACE: Geriatric Resources for Assessment and Care of Elders[65]
- INTERACT: Interventions to Reduce Acute Care Transfers[66]

Data from Refs.[58–66]

---

gait problems, vision problems, medications that cause lightheadedness, environmental hazards, and chronic medical conditions (ie, stroke, arthritis). The first step in fall prevention is engagement of the older adult in exercise programs that focus on balance, strength, and flexibility. Additional steps advocated by NCOA are outlined in **Box 7**.[68]

Aging is often associated with changes in driving ability as vision, hearing, physical abilities, and cognitive changes impact the ability to drive safely. The National Highway Traffic Safety Administration (NHTSA) serves as the national coordinating agency for comprehensive older driver safety program guidelines and resources for older drivers and their caregivers.[69] The NHTSA provides guidelines for state-level programs, as well as resources for older adults and their caregivers related to safe driving. Guidelines for caregivers urge open dialogue with older adults about safe driving, including observations by families and friends and self-assessment. The decision to refrain from driving is often emotional and represents a stage of aging that is difficult to accept. Sensitivity and compassion by caregivers are integral, underscored by concern for safety. Once a decision to no longer drive is made by older individuals, NHTSA encourages development of a mobility action plan that addresses the

---

Box 6
Strategies to reduce hospital readmissions

- Engage key stakeholders
- Develop a comprehensive transition plan
- Enhance medication reconciliation and management
- Institute daily interdisciplinary communication
- Standardize plans, procedures, and forms
- Always send discharge summaries
- Give patients discharge plans that are easy to understand
- Follow up and coordinate support

Data from Li J, Young R, Williams MV. Optimizing transitions of care to reduce rehospitalizations. Cleve Clin J Med 2014;81(5):317–8; and Hansen LO, Young RS, Hinami K, et al. Interventions to reduce 30-day rehospitalization: a systematic review. Ann Intern Med 2011;155(8):520–28.

Box 7
Steps to reduce risk of falls in older adults (National Council on Aging)

- Engage older adult in programs to build balance, strength, and flexibility
- Discuss current health conditions
- Get vision and hearing checked annually
- Review medications with a doctor or pharmacist
- Perform a walk-through safety assessment of the home
  - Lighting
  - Stairs
  - Bathrooms
- Talk to family members and enlist support from others

Adapted from National Council on Aging. 6 steps to protect your older loved one from a fall. Available at: http://www.ncoa.org/improve-health/falls-prevention/6-steps-to-protect-your-older.html. Accessed November 2, 2014.

---

following needs: (1) routine errands, (2) regular educational, social, or religious events, and (3) community and social events.[69] Ultimately, safe driving entails not only the safety of the older adult, but road safety of others.

SUMMARY

Traumatic injury in older adults is a significant public-health issue with the potential to impact a broad segment of the US population in the coming decades. Life expectancy has increased, and rising numbers of older adults are impacted by injury. Ensuing challenges compel both researchers and clinicians to optimize management of this vulnerable population. This review has addressed several relevant areas of focus, including epidemiology, evidence-based management, and injury prevention. Special attention is given to cognitive and physical function impairments (frailty), transitions of care, and advanced care planning. Continued attention to these aspects of geriatric trauma, using a patient-centered approach, will not only guide providers in optimal management of patients, but may guide policymakers toward evidence-based decisions that will impact older adults for generations to come.

REFERENCES

1. Vincent GK, Velkoff VA. The next four decades, the older population in the United States: 2010 to 2050. Current population reports. Washington, DC: U.S. Department of Commerce, Economics and Statistics Administration, U.S. Census Bureau; 2010. p. 1.
2. Agency for Healthcare Research and Quality (AHRQ). Healthcare Cost and Utilization Project (HCUPnet). 2012. Available at: http://hcupnet.ahrq.gov. Accessed October 23, 2014.
3. American College of Surgeons (ACS). National trauma data bank 2013 annual report. Available at: https://www.facs.org/~/media/files/quality%20programs/trauma/ntdb/ntdb%20annual%20report%202013.ashx. Accessed September 20, 2014.

4. Centers for Disease Control and Prevention. Injury prevention and control: data and statistics (WISQARTM). Available at: http://www.cdc.gov/injury/wisqars/. Accessed September 15, 2014.

5. Acierno R, Hernandez MA, Amstadter AB, et al. Prevalence and correlates of emotional, physical, sexual, and financial abuse and potential neglect in the United States: the National Elder Mistreatment Study. Am J Public Health 2010;100(2):292.

6. Yelon JA, Luchette FA, editors. Geriatric trauma and critical care. 1st edition. New York: Springer; 2014.

7. American College of Surgeons (ACS) Committee on Trauma. Resources for optimal care of the injured patient. Chicago, IL: American College of Surgeons; 6th edition. 2014.

8. American College of Surgeons (ACS). Advanced trauma life support. Available at: https://www.facs.org/quality%20programs/trauma/atls. Accessed September 15, 2014.

9. Emergency Nurses Association. Trauma nurse core course. Available at: http://www.ena.org/education/ENPC-TNCC/tncc/Pages/aboutcourse.aspx. Accessed September 20, 2014.

10. Eastern Association for the Surgery of Trauma (EAST). Evaluation and management of geriatric trauma. Available at: http://www.east.org/resources/treatment-guidelines/geriatric-trauma,-evaluation-and-management-of. Accessed September 20, 2014.

11. Kerwin AJ, Haut ER, Burns JB, et al. The Eastern Association of the Surgery of Trauma approach to practice management guideline development using Grading of Recommendations, Assessment, Development, and Evaluation (GRADE) methodology. J Trauma Acute Care Surg 2012;73(5):S283–7.

12. Calland JF, Ingraham AM, Martin N, et al. Evaluation and management of geriatric trauma: an Eastern Association for the Surgery of Trauma practice management guideline. J Trauma Acute Care Surg 2012;73(5):S345–50.

13. American College of Surgeons (ACS). Trauma quality improvement program. Available at: https://www.facs.org/quality-programs/trauma/tqip. Accessed September 20, 2014.

14. Goodmanson NW, Rosengart MR, Barnato AE, et al. Defining geriatric trauma: when does age make a difference? Surgery 2012;152(4):668–75.

15. Hsia RY, Wang E, Saynina O, et al. Factors associated with trauma center use for elderly patients with trauma: a statewide analysis, 1999-2008. Arch Surg 2011; 146(5):585–92.

16. Rzepka SG, Malangoni MA, Rimm AA. Geriatric trauma hospitalization in the United States: a population-based study. J Clin Epidemiol 2001;54(6): 627–33.

17. Scheetz LJ. Trauma center versus non-trauma center admissions in adult trauma victims by age and gender. Prehosp Emerg Care 2004;8(3):268–72.

18. Rogers A, Rogers F, Bradburn E, et al. Old and undertriaged: a lethal combination. Am Surg 2012;78(6):711–5.

19. Mosenthal AC, Lavery RF, Addis M, et al. Isolated traumatic brain injury: age is an independent predictor of mortality and early outcome. J Trauma 2002;52(5): 907–11.

20. Kohn MA, Hammel JM, Bretz SW, et al. Trauma team activation criteria as predictors of patient disposition from the emergency department. Acad Emerg Med 2004;11(1):1–9.

21. Fallon WF Jr, Rader E, Zyzanski S, et al. Geriatric outcomes are improved by a geriatric trauma consultation service. J Trauma 2006;61(5):1040–6.

22. Franko J, Kish KJ, O'Connell BG, et al. Advanced age and preinjury warfarin anti-coagulation increase the risk of mortality after head trauma. J Trauma 2006;61(1): 107–10.
23. Pieracci FM, Eachempati SR, Shou J, et al. Degree of anticoagulation, but not warfarin use itself, predicts adverse outcomes after traumatic brain injury in elderly trauma patients. J Trauma 2007;63(3):525–30.
24. Ohm C, Mina A, Howells G, et al. Effects of antiplatelet agents on outcomes for elderly patients with traumatic intracranial hemorrhage. J Trauma 2005;58(3):518–22.
25. Neideen T, Lam M, Brasel KJ. Preinjury beta blockers are associated with increased mortality in geriatric trauma patients. J Trauma 2008;65(5): 1016–20.
26. Min L, Burruss S, Morley E, et al. A simple clinical risk nomogram to predict mortality-associated geriatric complications in severely-injured geriatric patients. J Trauma Acute Care Surg 2013;74(4):1125.
27. Min L, Ubhayakar N, Saliba D, et al. The vulnerable elders survey-13 predicts hospital complications and mortality in older adults with traumatic injury: a pilot study. J Am Geriatr Soc 2011;59(8):1471–6.
28. Joseph B, Pandit V, Zangbar B, et al. Superiority of frailty over age in predicting outcomes among geriatric trauma patients: a prospective analysis. JAMA Surg 2014;149:766–72.
29. Maxwell CA. Screening hospitalized injured older adults for cognitive impairment and pre-injury functional impairment. Appl Nurs Res 2013;26(3):146–50.
30. Clegg A, Young J, Iliffe S, et al. Frailty in elderly people. Lancet 2013;381(9868): 752–62.
31. Morley JE, Vellas B, Abellan van Kan G, et al. Frailty consensus: a call to action. J Am Med Dir Assoc 2013;14(6):392–7.
32. Maxwell CA, Mion LC, Mukherjee K, et al. Feasibility of screening for pre-injury frailty in hospitalized injured older adults. J Trauma Acute Care Surg 2015 Mar 4. [Epub ahead of print].
33. Saliba D, Elliott M, Rubenstein LZ, et al. The vulnerable elders survey: a tool for identifying vulnerable older people in the community. J Am Geriatr Soc 2001; 49(12):1691–9.
34. Collin C, Wade DT, Davies S, et al. The Barthel ADL index: a reliability study. Int Disabil Stud 1988;10(2):61–3.
35. Baker PS, Bodner EV, Allman RM. Measuring life-space mobility in community-dwelling older adults. J Am Geriatr Soc 2003;51(11):1610–4.
36. Katz S. Assessing self-maintenance: activities of daily living, mobility, and instru-mental activities of daily living. J Am Geriatr Soc 1983;31:721–7.
37. Rockwood K, Song X, MacKnight C, et al. A global clinical measure of fitness and frailty in elderly people. Can Med Assoc J 2005;173(5):489–95.
38. Subra J, Gillette-Guyonnet S, Cesari M, et al. The integration of frailty into clinical practice: preliminary results from the Gérontopôle. J Nutr Health Aging 2012; 16(8):714–20.
39. van Kan GA, Rolland YM, Morley JE, et al. Frailty: toward a clinical definition. J Am Med Dir Assoc 2008;9(2):71–2.
40. Fried LP, Tangen CM, Walston J, et al. Frailty in older adults: evidence for a phenotype. J Gerontol A Biol Sci Med Sci 2001;56(3):M146–56.
41. Campanelli CM. American Geriatrics Society updated beers criteria for poten-tially inappropriate medication use in older adults: the American Geriatrics Society 2012 Beers Criteria Update Expert Panel. J Am Geriatr Soc 2012; 60(4):616.

42. Carrier FM, Turgeon AF, Nicole PC, et al. Effect of epidural analgesia in patients with traumatic rib fractures: a systematic review and meta-analysis of randomized controlled trials. Can J Anaesth 2009;56(3):230–42.
43. Plassman BL, Langa KM, McCammon RJ, et al. Incidence of dementia and cognitive impairment, not dementia in the United States. Ann Neurol 2011;70(3):418–26.
44. Siddiqi N, House AO, Holmes JD. Occurrence and outcome of delirium in medical in-patients: a systematic literature review. Age Ageing 2006;35(4):350–64.
45. Ryan DJ, O'Regan NA, Caoimh RÓ, et al. Delirium in an adult acute hospital population: predictors, prevalence and detection. BMJ Open 2013;3 [pii:e001772].
46. Inouye SK, Van Dyck CH, Alessi CA, et al. Clarifying confusion: the confusion assessment method: a new method for detection of delirium. Ann Intern Med 1990;113(12):941–8.
47. Ely EW, Inouye SK, Bernard GR, et al. Delirium in mechanically ventilated patients: validity and reliability of the confusion assessment method for the intensive care unit (CAM-ICU). JAMA 2001;286(21):2703–10.
48. Wade CE, Kozar RA, Dyer CB, et al. Evaluation of nutrition deficits in adult and elderly trauma patients. J Parenter Enteral Nutr 2014 Feb 21. [Epub ahead of print].
49. Doig GS, Heighes PT, Simpson F, et al. Early enteral nutrition, provided within 24 h of injury or intensive care unit admission, significantly reduces mortality in critically ill patients: a meta-analysis of randomised controlled trials. Intensive Care Med 2009;35(12):2018–27.
50. Anbar R, Beloosesky Y, Cohen J, et al. Tight calorie control in geriatric patients following hip fracture decreases complications: a randomized, controlled study. Clin Nutr 2014;33(1):23–8.
51. Mosenthal AC, Murphy PA, Barker LK, et al. Changing the culture around end-of-life care in the trauma intensive care unit. J Trauma Acute Care Surg 2008;64(6): 1587–93.
52. Sudore RL, Schillinger D, Knight SJ, et al. Uncertainty about advance care planning treatment preferences among diverse older adults. J Health Commun 2010; 15(S2):159–71.
53. Jencks SF, Williams MV, Coleman EA. Rehospitalizations among patients in the Medicare fee-for-service program. N Engl J Med 2009;360(14):1418–28.
54. Mor V, Intrator O, Feng Z, et al. The revolving door of rehospitalization from skilled nursing facilities. Health Aff (Millwood) 2010;29(1):57–64.
55. Coleman E, Fox P. Managing patient care transitions: a report of the HMO Care Management Workgroup. Healthplan 2003;45:36–9.
56. Li J, Young R, Williams MV. Optimizing transitions of care to reduce rehospitalizations. Cleve Clin J Med 2014;81(5):312–20.
57. Hansen LO, Young RS, Hinami K, et al. Interventions to reduce 30-day rehospitalization: a systematic review. Ann Intern Med 2011;155(8):520–8.
58. Society of Hospital Medicine. Project BOOST: better outcomes by optimizing safe transitions. Available at: http://www.hospitalmedicine.org/BOOST/. Accessed November 2, 2014.
59. Boston University Medical Center. Project RED: re-engineered discharge. 2014. Available at: http://www.bu.edu/fammed/projectred/. Accessed November 2, 2014.
60. Institute for Healthcare Improvement. STAAR: state action on avoidable rehospitalizations. Available at: http://www.ihi.org/engage/Initiatives/completed/STAAR/Pages/default.aspx. Accessed November 2, 2014.
61. University of Colorado Denver. The Care transitions Program. Available at: http://www.caretransitions.org/. Accessed November 2, 2014.

62. Penn Nursing Science. Transitional Care Model. Available at: http://www.nursing. upenn.edu/media/transitionalcare/Pages/default.aspx. Accessed November 2, 2014.
63. The Illinois Transitional Care Consortium. The bridge Model. Available at: http:// www.transitionalcare.org/the-bridge-model/. Accessed November 2, 2014.
64. Johns Hopkins Bloomberg School of Public Health. Guided care. Available at: http://www.jhsph.edu/research/centers-and-institutes/roger-c-lipitz-center-for-integrated-health-care/Guided_Care/. Accessed November 2, 2014.
65. Counsell SR, Callahan CM, Buttar AB, et al. Geriatric Resources for Assessment and Care of Elders (GRACE): a new model of primary care for low-income seniors. J Am Geriatr Soc 2006;54(7):1136–41.
66. Florida Atlantic University. INTERACT: interventions to reduce acute care transfers. Available at: http://interact2.net/. Accessed November 2, 2014.
67. Centers for Disease Control and Prevention. Costs of falls among older adults. 2014. Available at: http://www.cdc.gov/homeandrecreationalsafety/falls/fallcost. html. Accessed October 23, 2014.
68. National Council on Aging (NCOA). 6 steps to protect your older loved one from a fall. Available at: http://www.ncoa.org/improve-health/falls-prevention/6-steps-to-protect-your-older.html. Accessed November 2, 2014.
69. National Highway Traffic Safety Administration (NHTSA). Older drivers. Available at: http://www.nhtsa.gov/Driving+Safety/Older+Drivers. Accessed November 2, 2014.

Trauma Resuscitation and Monitoring

Military Lessons Learned

Elizabeth J. Bridges, PhD, RN, CCNS[a],*,
Margaret M. McNeill, PhD, RN, APRN-CNS, CCRN, CCNS, NE-BC, CIP[b,c]

KEYWORDS

- Monitoring/physiologic • Combat casualty care • Military medicine • Wounds
- Injuries

KEY POINTS

- Systolic blood pressure (SBP) and heart rate (HR) are not sensitive indicators of hypoperfusion.
- Hypoperfusion may begin with an SBP of 100 to 110 mm Hg.
- Shock index is a more sensitive and specific indicator of hypoperfusion than SBP or HR alone.
- New dynamic, noninvasive monitors may provide earlier and more sensitive indications of deterioration or occult hypoperfusion.

The management of a patient with a severe injury requires careful resuscitation and astute monitoring. The principles of trauma management have evolved over the past several years, partly due to the military experiences in the care of casualties in Iraq and Afghanistan.[1] The United States and coalition partners have demonstrated an unprecedented reduction in combat-related deaths, despite an increase in injury severity. Within the context of a 7000-mile-long continuum of care from the point of injury to the United States and the new practices associated with damage-control resuscitation, this article draws on military research regarding the limitations of current vital sign monitoring and introduces innovative monitoring technologies that may be beneficial in severely injured patients.

The authors have nothing to disclose.
[a] Biobehavioral Nursing and Health Systems, University of Washington School of Nursing, Box 357266, Seattle, WA 98195, USA; [b] University of Washington Medical Center, Seattle, WA, USA; [c] Department of Professional and Clinical Development, Frederick Memorial Hospital, 400 West Seventh Street, Frederick, MD 21701, USA
* Corresponding author.
E-mail address: ebridges@u.washington.edu

MILITARY TRAUMA CARE ACROSS THE CONTINUUM

The Joint Theater Trauma System (JTTS) was developed with the vision that every soldier, marine, sailor, and airman injured on the battlefield will have the optimal chance for survival and maximum potential for functional recovery. The military trauma care continuum begins at the point of injury and extends to definitive care in the United States (**Fig. 1**).[2] In this system, medical capabilities are as close to the battlefield as possible,[3] resulting in the need to provide critical care, including damage-control resuscitation, during transport for the patients.[4,5] Global en route care and the Air Force Critical Care Air Transport Teams (CCATTs) have revolutionized combat critical care. The CCATTs, with a critical care physician, nurse, and respiratory therapist, transport patients in a cargo aircraft on missions that range from 1 to 18 hours, with most flights 6 to 8 hours long.[6] During the Vietnam War, patients were evacuated from theater to a remote hospital in 21 days; with the CCATTs, the average time to transport after an injury is 28 hours, and often as little as 12 hours.[3] Rapid movement of critically injured casualties (average Injury Severity Score 23.7) within hours of wounding is safe, with a minimal mortality during movement (0.02%). These patients have a 30-day mortality (2.1%) that is independent of the time from injury to arrival at definitive care.[7] Among 1491 patients transported by CCATT, 69% suffered polytrauma, primarily due to explosions. The injuries are complex, including soft tissue trauma (64%), orthopedic (45%), thoracic (35%), skull fracture (27%), and brain injuries (25%).[8] These patients, who may be stabilizing but not stable, require ongoing interventions and monitoring during the en route phase of care, which is challenging given the austere and dynamic conditions onboard an aircraft. The integration of new research and practice on the battlefield and during transport, and a system to support care across the 7000-mile continuum from the battlefield to the United States, has been instrumental in the unprecedented survival rate for combat casualties.[9–12]

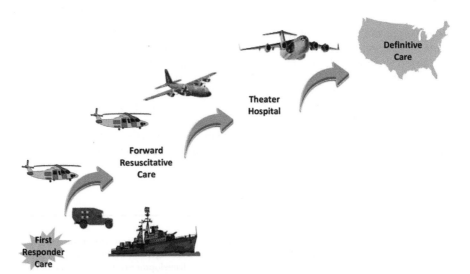

Fig. 1. Military en route care continuum. The US military en route care system begins at the point of injury and extends to definitive care in the United States. Along the continuum, care is provided at military trauma hospitals and by highly specialized transport teams onboard military ground, sea, and air transports. (*Adapted from* Chairman Joint Chiefs of Staff (CJCS). Health service support (Joint Publication 4–02). 2012. Available at: http://www.dtic.mil/doctrine/new_pubs/jp4_02.pdf. Accessed November 15, 2014.)

THE GOAL OF TRAUMA RESUSCITATION: CONTROL THE TRAUMA TRIAD

Traumatic injuries may result in death or severe disability unless the trauma team is able to control life-threatening complications known as the Trauma Triad of Death: hypothermia, acidosis, and coagulopathy.[13] In trauma patients, even after controlling for injury severity and other confounders, hypothermia remains an independent predictor of mortality (odds ratio [OR]1.19; 95% confidence interval [CI] 1.05–1.35),[14] with mortality associated with hypothermia-associated coagulopathy and inflammatory effects.[15] Severe acidosis (eg, pH <7.1 or a base deficit of −12.5 mmol/L or less) also impairs hemostasis. The third aspect of the Triad of Death is coagulopathy. Uncontrolled hemorrhage remains the leading cause of battlefield deaths, and the second cause of early death after civilian trauma,[16–20] although the use of prehospital extremity tourniquets has improved survival in combat casualties.[21]

Acute traumatic coagulopathy (ATC), which is an endogenous impairment of all components of hemostasis, is related to injury severity and shock, and is associated with poor outcomes.[22] ATC develops rapidly and has been identified within minutes of injury.[23] Rather than merely a consumptive coagulopathy, ATC is characterized by isolated factor V inhibition, dysfibrinogenemia, systemic anticoagulation, impaired platelet function, and hyperfibrinolysis. ATC is exacerbated by continued blood loss, hypothermia, acidosis, and resuscitation with hypocoagulable fluids, which contribute collectively to establish trauma-induced coagulopathy (TIC).[23,24] TIC management includes replacement of coagulation factors along with packed red blood cells (PRBCs) in the form of a massive transfusion protocol. Adjuncts may include tranexamic acid, recombinant factor VIIa (rFVIIa), and fibrinogen replacement.[25]

MASSIVE TRANSFUSION PROTOCOLS AND DAMAGE-CONTROL RESUSCITATION

Massive transfusion, a form of hemostatic resuscitation, is one component of damage-control resuscitation (DCR) (**Box 1**).[1,26] The exsanguinating patient requiring massive transfusion is at significant risk of death from uncontrolled bleeding and persistent coagulopathy.[27] Early recognition of the patient requiring a massive transfusion (10 or more units of PRBCs within 24 hours), is essential (**Box 2**).[28,29] The JTTS developed Clinical Practice Guidelines (CPGs) related to the various aspects of DCR, including hypothermia prevention and massive transfusions.[30] Since the 2006 implementation of these CPGs, along with a dramatic "revolution" in operational military medical care, the case fatality rate decreased from 17% to 8% in 2013, despite an increase in injury severity.[9,11]

Box 1
Tenets of damage-control resuscitation

- Body rewarming
- Correction of acidosis
- Permissive hypotension
- Restrictive fluid administration
- Early diagnosis of coagulopathy
- Hemostatic resuscitation

Data from Davis DT, Johannigman JA, Pritts TA. New strategies for massive transfusion in the bleeding trauma patient. J Trauma Nurs 2012;19:69–75; and Kaafarani HM, Velmahos GC. Damage control resuscitation. Scand J Surg 2014;103:81–8.

Box 2
Predictors for massive transfusion in severely injured patients

- SBP <110 mm Hg
- HR >105 beats per minute
- Hematocrit <32%
- pH <7.25

Patients with 3 of the above 4 factors have an approximately 70% predicted risk of massive transfusion; patients with all 4 have an 85% predicted risk.

- Other risk factors include international normalized ratio >1.4, skeletal tissue oxygenation <75%[29]

Data from Schreiber MA, Perkins J, Kiraly L, et al. Early predictors of massive transfusion in combat casualties. J Am Coll Surg 2007;205:541–5; and Moore FA, Nelson T, McKinley BA, et al. Massive transfusion in trauma patients: tissue hemoglobin oxygen saturation predicts poor outcome. J Trauma 2008;64:1010–23.

Recent military experience supports DCR.[31,32] Central to DCR is aggressive management with predefined ratios of plasma to PRBCs.[1] The DCR approach recommends earlier and more balanced transfusion of plasma and platelets along with the first units of RBCs (ie, maintaining plasma:platelet:RBC ratios closer to the 1:1:1 ratio of whole blood), while minimizing crystalloid use.[33] Higher plasma and platelet ratios early in resuscitation are associated with decreased mortality in patients who received at least 3 units of blood products during the first 24 hours after admission.[34] Among survivors at 24 hours, the subsequent risk of 30-day mortality was not associated with plasma or platelet ratios.

Although surgical and angio-intervention techniques remain the cornerstone for the management of severe bleeding after trauma, adjunct therapeutic strategies, such as local or systemic hemostatic agents, can play an important role.[35] The aim of any hemostatic therapy is to control bleeding and minimize blood loss and transfusion requirements.[36] Two agents used by both the military and civilian trauma teams in the treatment of uncontrolled hemorrhage are rFVIIa and tranexamic acid (TXA). Evidence supporting the use of rFVIIa is equivocal, with military and civilian studies finding that rFVIIa was neither associated with improved survival nor an increase in complications.[37,38] A limitation of both military and civilian studies has been the lack of clear identification of which severely injured patients require or may benefit from rFVIIa.[39] In contrast, in both civilian and military trauma, early administration of TXA is associated with decreased mortality and risk of death due to bleeding.[40,41] In a Cochrane review of 2 trials (n = 20,451), TXA reduced the risk of death by 10% (relative risk [RR] 0.90, 95% CI 0.85–0.97; P = .0035) and in one trial involving 20,211 patients, TXA decreased the risk of death due to bleeding by 15% (RR 0.85, 95% CI 0.76–0.96; P = .0077). There is evidence that early treatment ($\leq$3 hours) is more effective than late treatment (>3 hours).[42]

In a study of 59 British military personnel who received massive transfusions, 85% survived to discharge from the hospital, and 5 of 7 patients who received greater than 100 units of blood products survived.[43] Keys to the success of DCR are the early identification of patients requiring DCR, a system to ensure the consistent use of evidence-based DCR strategies, and the capability to safely transport these critically injured patients to definitive care.

HEMODYNAMIC MONITORING

Critical to improving outcomes for severely injured patients is the rapid identification of high-risk patients, the initiation of life-saving interventions (LSIs), and monitoring during DCR to ensure the resolution of hypoperfusion. A challenge is that routine vital signs (heart rate [HR], systolic blood pressure [SBP]) are not sensitive or specific indicators of clinical deterioration. This section addresses evidence about the use of vital signs in trauma (**Box 3**) and newer "vital signs" for identifying high-risk individuals.

VITAL SIGNS

Advanced Trauma Life Support (ATLS) classifies the severity of shock based on HR, SBP, pulse pressure (PP), respiratory rate, mental status, and urine output.[47] The thresholds traditionally considered indicative of the onset of hypoperfusion (SBP ≤90 mm Hg and HR >120 beats per minute) are not supported by strong evidence. Although the HR does increase and the SBP does decrease with increasing blood loss, they do not change to the extent outlined in the ATLS guidelines.[48] For example, in a study of data from 165,785 trauma patients, among 121,646 patients with Class I shock (<15% estimated blood loss), the median HR and SBP were 82 beats per minute and 135 mm Hg, respectively. However, in 8984 patients with Class IV shock (>40% estimated blood loss), the median HR was 95 beats per minute and the median SBP was 120 mm Hg, which are also consistent with Class I shock. This study demonstrates that sole reliance on the HR and SBP underestimates the severity of the blood loss. In severely injured combat victims with hemorrhagic shock but no head injury, there was no difference in field vital signs or SpO$_2$ between casualties who lived or died.[49] An increase in the HR can be caused by numerous factors, the SBP is often maintained in a normal range until acute decompensation occurs, and patients requiring LSIs may still have normal vital signs.[45]

If occult hypoperfusion persists, an oxygen debt can develop, which is associated with increased morbidity and mortality. In 48 critically injured patients, there

---

Box 3
Evidence related to standard vital sign monitoring in trauma

Systolic Blood Pressure (SBP)

- Hypoperfusion may begin with an SBP of 100–110 mm Hg

- The SBP at which hypoperfusion begins is higher in adults older than 43 years (117 mm Hg) in contrast to younger individuals (108 mm Hg)[44]

Shock Index (SI)

- The SI is a more sensitive and specific indicator of hypoperfusion than the heart rate (HR) or SBP alone

- An SI ≥0.9 is indicative of hypoperfusion; however, an SI can be normal in cases of occult hypoperfusion and should not be used as the sole indicator of hypoperfusion

- An increase in the SI >0.3 may indicate occult blood loss (ie, blood loss with hypoperfusion despite a normal SBP and HR)

- In patients with normal vital signs, the addition of the SI does not identify patients in need of life-saving interventions[45]

- The SI may be attenuated in cases of moderate to severe traumatic brain injury[46]

Data from Refs.[44–46]

was no significant difference in the mean arterial pressure (MAP) between survivors and nonsurvivors, and in both groups, the MAP was within normal limits. Both groups were tachycardic, with nonsurvivors having a higher HR. In contrast to the nonpredictive changes in the MAP and HR, there was a significant difference in tissue perfusion, as indicated by transcutaneous oxygen ($P_{tc}O_2$) and carbon dioxide levels ($P_{tc}CO_2$). The nonsurvivors had lower $P_{tc}O_2$ values and higher $P_{tc}CO_2$ compared with survivors. The survivors who developed organ failure had longer periods of hypoperfusion compared with survivors who did not develop organ failure (31 vs 5 minutes and 17 vs 1 minute, respectively). Patients with more than 60 minutes of decreased tissue perfusion had a mortality of 89% and a 100% incidence of organ failure or sepsis.[50] This study highlights that even short periods of hypoperfusion increase the risk for multisystem organ failure and death and, given the limitations of standard vital signs and intermittent laboratory values, emphasizes the need for more sensitive, real-time measures to assess a patient's perfusion status.

Systolic Blood Pressure

A common assumption is that an SBP less than 90 mm Hg is the threshold for the onset of hypoperfusion. In a study of data from 870,634 patients in the National Trauma Data Bank, the onset of hypoperfusion, as indicated by an increase in base deficit above baseline, occurred when the SBP decreased below 118 mm Hg and mortality increased 6% for every 10 mm Hg decrease in SBP below 115 mm Hg.[44] When the SBP was 90 mm Hg, the average base deficit was −8 mmol/L, indicating moderately severe occult hypoperfusion despite a "normal" SBP. Similar results were found in 7180 military combat trauma casualties.[51] In these patients, the base deficit began to increase when the SBP decreased below 100 mm Hg, and the mortality increased by 4% with an admission SBP of 90 to 100 mm Hg compared with patients with an admission SBP of 101 to 110 mm Hg.

Shock Index

The shock index (SI), which is the ratio of HR to SBP (SI = HR/BP), is inversely related to blood loss, cardiac index, stroke volume, MAP, left ventricular stroke work, and oxygen delivery.[52] In general, an SI ≥ 0.9 is considered abnormal, thus any time the HR is greater than the SBP, the SI will be abnormal, and further evaluation of the patient is warranted. For example, if a patient has an HR of 120 and an SBP of 100 mm Hg, the SI is 1.2 beats per mm Hg. More specific SI ranges,[53,54] which are consistent with increasing base deficit (sp) and lactate, are as follows:

- SI <0.6 (no shock)
- SI ≥ 0.6 to <1.0 (mild shock)
- SI ≥ 1.0 to <1.4 (moderate shock)
- SI ≥ 1.4 (severe shock)

The SI is a more accurate indicator of hypoperfusion than HR or SBP alone. Studies published in the 1990s found an increase in the SI and continued hypoperfusion in patients with a variety of causes of shock (eg, septic, cardiogenic, hemorrhagic), despite normalization of the HR and SBP.[55,56] In healthy blood donors (450 mL), the SI increased from normal to abnormal (>0.7), despite a normal HR and SBP.[57] These studies reiterate the limitations of SBP and HR as independent indicators of blood loss and hypoperfusion, in contrast to SI, which may be sensitive to a relatively small blood loss.

A higher SI on admission to the emergency department (ED) is associated with increased base deficit and lactate, indicating poorer perfusion. In 21,853 trauma patients, individuals with an admission SI less than 0.6 had a normal lactate (2.7 ± 1.7 mmol/L) in contrast to patients with severe shock (SI ≥1.4), who had a lactate of 6.0 ± 8.4.[53] Of note, in this study, the SBP decreased with increasing SI, but on average the SBP was never less than 90 mm Hg, even with an SI greater than or equal to 1.4, demonstrating the benefit of the SI over the SBP as an indication of hypoperfusion.

An increased SI (>0.9) is associated with an increased risk of mortality. Trauma patients with an ED SI greater than 0.9 had a mortality of 15.9% compared with a 6.3% mortality rate in patients with an ED SI less than 0.9. The trend in the SI is also important. A change in the SI of 0.3 or more from prehospital to the ED was associated with an increased mortality (27.6%) compared with 5.8% mortality in patients with a change in SI less than 0.3.[58] The SI also may be useful as part of secondary (in-hospital) triage. In 485 combat trauma patients, an SI greater than or equal to 0.75 on ED admission adequately identified patients who required LSIs, such as intubation, blood products, or emergent surgery,[59] and has been used to evaluate a change in perfusion status during transport.[60]

NEWER VITAL SIGNS

Assessment of combat casualties in the field is focused on triage and the identification of patients who require LSIs.[44] Despite the potential utility of a minimal vital sign set (eg, radial pulse characteristics, Glasgow Coma Scale [GCS]) to identify patients requiring prehospital LSIs,[61–64] vital signs alone may fail to identify occult hypoperfusion.[65] Recently, military and civilian researchers have demonstrated the potential utility of noninvasive continuous monitoring to detect hypoperfusion and guide resuscitative therapy.

Wireless Vital Signs Monitor: Murphy Factor

Recent research suggests acute changes in vital signs may be more predictive of the need for LSIs than isolated vital signs. A wireless vital signs monitor developed by US Special Operations Command collects and transmits any available vital sign data and calculates an acuity algorithm based on the vital signs changes over the preceding 30 seconds (Murphy Factor). The Murphy Factor was better at predicting the need for an LSI on admission to the hospital (area under the curve 0.62) compared with an HR greater than 100 beats per minute, SBP less than 90 mm Hg, or oxygen saturation (SaO2) less than 95% (alone or in combination).[66]

Compensatory Reserve Index

The Compensatory Reserve Index (CRI) is obtained by the automated analysis of changes in the shape of a pulse oximeter waveform (photoplethysmography),[67,68] which reflects the compensatory cardiopulmonary response to loss of central circulating volume (eg, hemorrhage). Monitoring these changes quantifies the amount of compensation remaining (ie, compensatory reserve) to respond to a further decrease in effective circulating volume, and to identify when a patient is on the verge of decompensation. The CRI is reported on a 0 to 1 scale, with a CRI of 1 indicating maximum compensation available, a CRI of 0.6 indicating that 40% of the compensatory reserve has been used ("moderate compromise") and a CRI of 0.3 indicating severe compromise and impending decompensation. A study[69] in 15 healthy subjects used lower body negative pressure (LBNP), which simulates hemorrhage. With progressive LBNP, the SI reached 0.9 or higher in approximately 22 minutes (at an LBNP that caused translocation of $\sim$1000 mL or more of blood from the central circulation and a 65% decrease in stroke volume [SV]). In contrast, a CRI of 0.6 ("moderate compromise") occurred 14 minutes earlier (at an LBNP causing 550–1000 mL blood translocation), and a CRI of 0.3 ("hemodynamic instability") occurred approximately 5 minutes before the SI reached 0.9 and the subject acutely decompensated (decrease SBP/increase HR). Thus, the CRI may provide an earlier warning of clinical deterioration.[69,70] An important finding is that on average, individuals can lose between 40% and 70% of their compensatory reserve before any change occurs in their HR, SBP, PP, or SI.

There is limited research on the use of the CRI in patients with acute hemorrhage. In healthy subjects donating 450 mL of blood, the CRI decreased from 0.74 before donation to 0.62 (16% decrease) in contrast to a 3% decrease in SBP (124–119 mm Hg), a 7% increase in SI (0.68–0.72) and a 2% increase in HR (83–85 beats per minute).[71] In these patients, a CRI of 0.6 had a sensitivity of 0.43 and a specificity of 0.97 to detect a minor (450 mL) blood loss, which means that a CRI of 0.6 or less very accurately identifies individuals who have suffered a minor blood loss (true positive); however, there were a large number of individuals with a CRI greater than 0.6 who suffered an undetected blood loss (false negative). Compared with routine vital signs, the CRI was a more accurate indicator of a minor blood loss. Further research is needed to define the appropriate thresholds in acutely bleeding trauma victims.

Near-Infrared Spectroscopy–Skeletal Tissue Oxygenation

Near-infrared spectroscopy technology has been used to noninvasively measure the percent saturation of skin or muscle tissue oxygenation, via a probe placed on the hand or forearm. Skeletal tissue oxygenation (StO_2) provides an indication of hypoperfusion independent of changes in the vital signs,[72–74] and it is highly correlated with oxygen delivery, base excess, and lactate.[75] The normal StO_2 is greater than 75% and an StO_2 less than 50% indicates hypoperfusion. In healthy subjects, the mean StO_2 was 87% $\pm$ 6%, and in trauma victims the StO_2 differentiated between severe shock and mild/moderate shock, but not between the absence of shock and mild or moderate shock.[76] A case series[77] of combat casualties demonstrated the potential utility of StO_2 to detect occult hypoperfusion. Among 40 casualties evaluated using StO_2, 8 (20%) had an initial StO_2 less than 70%. **Table 1** summarizes the initial presentation of 4 of these patients. Of note, in the first 2 cases the StO_2 identifies physiologic deterioration (low StO_2) despite normal vital signs (occult hypoperfusion), and in the remaining 2 patients, the StO_2 confirms the severity of the hypoperfusion.

Beekley[78] studied the ability of StO_2 to predict the need for an LSI in 147 combat casualties. The patients who required an LSI had a significantly lower StO_2 compared

Table 1 StO_2 monitoring in combat casualties			
Patient Injury	**BP**	**HR**	**StO_2**
IED Blast with bilateral amputations	110/70	110	51%
GSW to abdomen	90/60	120	50%
High velocity GSW to hip: on 100% O_2	56/30	150	54%
IED blast with massive right lower extremity injury, SaO_2 91%	69	150	52%

Abbreviations: BP, blood pressure; GSW, gunshot wound; HR, heart rate; IED, improvised explosive device; StO_2, skeletal tissue oxygenation.

Data from Beilman GJ, Blondet JJ. Tissue oxygen saturation in battlefield injuries using near-infrared spectroscopy: a case series report. World J Emerg Surg 2009;4:25.

with patients who did not require an LSI, blood transfusion, or a massive transfusion. Of interest, in the 132 of 147 casualties with an admission SBP greater than 90 mm Hg (theoretically at risk for occult hypoperfusion), the only independent predictors of a need for a blood transfusion were StO_2 (OR 1.35) and hematocrit (OR 2.66). These results are similar to a recent study in 325 rural trauma patients, where an ED StO_2 less than 65% was associated with greater blood transfusion requirements over the next 24 hours.[79] In a recent case series, StO_2 was obtained on the battlefield at the point of injury.[80] The first StO_2 (and vital signs) were obtained 22 ± 7 minutes after the injury. Five of 6 casualties had severe extremity trauma requiring tourniquets and 1 casualty suffered a bowel evisceration after being hit by a rocket. At the point of injury, 2 patients were hypoperfused (SBP <90 mm Hg), both with StO_2 less than 75%, and on arrival to Combat Support Hospital, both patients had moderate/severe increase in lactate. In 2 other patients, the field StO_2 did not identify the mild increase in lactate noted on arrival to the hospital, and the StO_2 was greater than 75% in 2 patients with normal lactate. In this small case series, an abnormal StO_2 (<75%) was indicative of hypoperfusion, independent of the vital signs, but a normal StO_2 (>75%) did not consistently detect mild or moderate hypoperfusion, which is similar to previous research. This observational study was extended to 48 severely injured combat casualties who were post-DCR and undergoing medical evacuation to a higher level of care. Before transport, 39 patients had base deficit, with hypoperfusion in 27 patients (21/27 occult, 5 moderate/severe hypoperfusion). In these patients, the StO_2 was poorly correlated with the base deficit, although it is unknown if the lack of correlation reflected the real-time StO_2 assessment of the patients' perfusion state in contrast to the base deficit, which could have been collected up to 5 hours before transport. The study highlights the need to identify real-time methods to assess perfusion status, rather than intermittent measurements as the patient moves across the care continuum. Recent trauma research suggests that a dynamic StO_2 measurement (rate of StO_2 decrease caused by vascular occlusion), which is thought to reflect local metabolic rate, may be predictive of in-hospital LSIs.[81]

SUMMARY

Over the past 13 years, the military health care system has made improvements that are associated with an unprecedented survival rate for severely injured casualties. Monitoring for indications of deterioration as the critically injured patient moves across the continuum of care is difficult given the limitations of routinely used vital signs. Research by both military and civilian researchers is revolutionizing monitoring, with an increased focus on noninvasive, continuous, dynamic measurements to provide earlier, more sensitive indications of the patient's perfusion status.

REFERENCES

1. Davis DT, Johannigman JA, Pritts TA. New strategies for massive transfusion in the bleeding trauma patient. J Trauma Nurs 2012;19:69–75.
2. Chairman Joint Chiefs of Staff (CJCS). Health service support (Joint Publication 4–02). 2012. Available at: http://www.dtic.mil/doctrine/new_pubs/jp4_02.pdf. Accessed November 15, 2014.
3. Johannigman JA. Maintaining the continuum of en route care. Crit Care Med 2008;36(7 Suppl):S377–82.
4. Davis RS, Connelly LK. Nursing and en route care: history in time of war. US Army Med Dep J 2011;45–50.

5. Mathews J. USAF's 'care in the air' exceeds expectations. Aviation Week & Space Technology. 2014. http://awin.aviationweek.com/portals/awin/Interactives/AWST/ERCCS/ERCCS.html. Accessed October 15, 2014.

6. Blackbourne LH, Baer DG, Eastridge BJ, et al. Military medical revolution: deployed hospital and en route care. J Trauma Acute Care Surg 2012; 73(6 Suppl 5):S378–87.

7. Ingalls N, Zonies D, Bailey JA, et al. A review of the first 10 years of critical care aeromedical transport during Operation Iraqi Freedom and Operation Enduring Freedom: the importance of evacuation timing. JAMA Surg 2014;149:807–13.

8. Bridges E, Evers K. Wartime critical care air transport. Mil Med 2009;174:370–5.

9. Blackbourne LH, Baer DG, Eastridge BJ, et al. Military medical revolution: military trauma system. J Trauma Acute Care Surg 2012;73(6 Suppl 5):S388–94.

10. Rasmussen TE. The military's evolved en route care paradigm: continuous, transcontinental intensive care. JAMA Surg 2014;149:814.

11. Rasmussen TE, Gross KR, Baer DG. Where do we go from here? Preface. US Military Health System Research Symposium, August 2013. J Trauma Acute Care Surg 2013;75(2 Suppl 2):S105–6.

12. McNeill MM. 7000 miles and 7 days from the battlefield. AACN Adv Crit Care 2010;21:307–15.

13. Mikhail J. The trauma triad of death: hypothermia, acidosis, and coagulopathy. AACN Clin Issues 1999;10:85–94.

14. Shafi S, Elliott AC, Gentilello L. Is hypothermia simply a marker of shock and injury severity or an independent risk factor for mortality in trauma patients? Analysis of a large national trauma registry. J Trauma 2005;59:1081–5.

15. Hildebrand F, Giannoudis PV, van Griensven M, et al. Pathophysiologic changes and effects of hypothermia on outcome in elective surgery and trauma patients. Am J Surg 2004;187:363–71.

16. Cothren CC, Moore EE, Hedegaard HB, et al. Epidemiology of urban trauma deaths: a comprehensive reassessment 10 years later. World J Surg 2007;31:1507–11.

17. Evans JA, van Wessem KJ, McDougall D, et al. Epidemiology of traumatic deaths: comprehensive population-based assessment. World J Surg 2010;34: 158–63.

18. Shackelford SA, Colton K, Stansbury LG, et al. Early identification of uncontrolled hemorrhage after trauma: current status and future direction. J Trauma Acute Care Surg 2014;77(3 Suppl 2):S222–2227.

19. Eastridge BJ, Mabry RL, Seguin P, et al. Death on the battlefield (2001–2011): implications for the future of combat casualty care. J Trauma Acute Care Surg 2012;73(6 Suppl 5):S431–7.

20. Champion HR, Bellamy RF, Roberts CP, et al. A profile of combat injury. J Trauma 2003;54(5 Suppl):S13–9.

21. Kragh JF Jr, Littrel ML, Jones JA, et al. Battle casualty survival with emergency tourniquet use to stop limb bleeding. J Emerg Med 2011;41:590–7.

22. Lamb CM, MacGoey P, Navarro AP, et al. Damage control surgery in the era of damage control resuscitation. Br J Anaesth 2014;113:242–9.

23. Frith D, Brohi K. The pathophysiology of trauma-induced coagulopathy. Curr Opin Crit Care 2012;18:631–6.

24. Davenport R. Pathogenesis of acute traumatic coagulopathy. Transfusion 2013; 53(Suppl 1):23S–7S.

25. Sharrock AE, Midwinter M. Damage control—trauma care in the first hour and beyond: a clinical review of relevant developments in the field of trauma care. Ann R Coll Surg Engl 2013;95:177–83.

26. Kaafarani HM, Velmahos GC. Damage control resuscitation. Scand J Surg 2014; 103:81–8.
27. Spinella PC, Holcomb JB. Resuscitation and transfusion principles for traumatic hemorrhagic shock. Blood Rev 2009;23:231–40.
28. Schreiber MA, Perkins J, Kiraly L, et al. Early predictors of massive transfusion in combat casualties. J Am Coll Surg 2007;205:541–5.
29. Moore FA, Nelson T, McKinley BA, et al. Massive transfusion in trauma patients: tissue hemoglobin oxygen saturation predicts poor outcome. J Trauma 2008;64: 1010–23.
30. US Army Institute of Surgical Research. JTS and CCATT Clinical Practice Guidelines. 2014. Available at: http://www.usaisr.amedd.army.mil/clinical_practice_guidelines.html. Accessed November 25, 2014.
31. Campion EM, Pritts TA, Dorlac WC, et al. Implementation of a military-derived damage-control resuscitation strategy in a civilian trauma center decreases acute hypoxia in massively transfused patients. J Trauma Acute Care Surg 2013;75(2 Suppl 2):S221–7.
32. Langan NR, Eckert M, Martin MJ. Changing patterns of in-hospital deaths following implementation of damage control resuscitation practices in US forward military treatment facilities. JAMA Surg 2014;149:904–12.
33. Holcomb JB, Pati S. Optimal trauma resuscitation with plasma as the primary resuscitative fluid: the surgeon's perspective. Hematology Am Soc Hematol Educ Program 2013;2013:656–9.
34. Holcomb JB, del Junco DJ, Fox EE, et al. The prospective, observational, multi-center, major trauma transfusion (PROMMTT) study: comparative effectiveness of a time-varying treatment with competing risks. JAMA Surg 2013;148:127–36.
35. Georgiou C, Neofytou K, Demetriades D. Local and systemic hemostatics as an adjunct to control bleeding in trauma. Am Surg 2013;79:180–7.
36. Fries D. The early use of fibrinogen, prothrombin complex concentrate, and recombinant-activated factor VIIa in massive bleeding. Transfusion 2013; 53(Suppl 1):91S–5S.
37. Wade CE, Eastridge BJ, Jones JA, et al. Use of recombinant factor VIIa in US military casualties for a five-year period. J Trauma Acute Care Surg 2010;69:353–9.
38. Hauser CJ, Boffard K, Dutton R, et al. Results of the CONTROL trial: efficacy and safety of recombinant activated Factor VII in the management of refractory traumatic hemorrhage. J Trauma Acute Care Surg 2010;69:489–500.
39. Knudson MM, Cohen MJ, Reidy R, et al. Trauma, transfusions, and use of recombinant factor VIIa: a multicenter case registry report of 380 patients from the Western Trauma Association. J Am Coll Surg 2011;212:87–95.
40. Shakur H, Roberts I, Bautista R, et al. Effects of tranexamic acid on death, vascular occlusive events, and blood transfusion in trauma patients with significant haemorrhage (CRASH-2): a randomised, placebo-controlled trial. Lancet 2010;376:23–32.
41. Morrison JJ, Dubose JJ, Rasmussen TE, et al. Military Application of Tranexamic Acid in Trauma Emergency Resuscitation (MATTERs) Study. Arch Surg 2012;147:113–9.
42. Roberts I, Shakur H, Ker K, et al. Antifibrinolytic drugs for acute traumatic injury. Cochrane Database Syst Rev 2012;(12):CD004896.
43. Allcock EC, Woolley T, Doughty H, et al. The clinical outcome of UK military personnel who received a massive transfusion in Afghanistan during 2009. J R Army Med Corps 2011;15:365–9.
44. Eastridge BJ, Salinas J, McManus JG, et al. Hypotension begins at 110 mm Hg: redefining "hypotension" with data. J Trauma 2007;63(2):291–7.

45. Convertino VA, Ryan KL, Rickards CA, et al. Physiological and medical monitoring for en route care of combat casualties. J Trauma 2008;64(4 Suppl):S342–53.

46. McMahon CG, Kenny R, Bennett K, et al. The effect of acute traumatic brain injury on the performance of shock index. J Trauma Acute Care Surg 2010;69: 1169–75.

47. American College of Surgeons. Advanced trauma life support for doctors. 9th edition. Chicago: American College of Surgeons; 2012.

48. Guly HR, Bouamra O, Spiers M, et al. Vital signs and estimated blood loss in patients with major trauma: testing the validity of the ATLS classification of hypovolaemic shock. Resuscitation 2011;82:556–9.

49. Cooke WH, Salinas J, Convertino VA, et al. Heart rate variability and its association with mortality in prehospital trauma patients. J Trauma 2006;60:363–70.

50. Tatevossian RG, Wo CC, Velmahos GC, et al. Transcutaneous oxygen and CO2 as early warning of tissue hypoxia and hemodynamic shock in critically ill emergency patients. Crit Care Med 2000;28:2248–53.

51. Eastridge BJ, Salinas J, Wade CE, et al. Hypotension is 100 mm Hg on the battlefield. Am J Surg 2011;202:404–8.

52. Rady MY, Nightingale P, Little RA, et al. Shock index: a re-evaluation in acute circulatory failure. Resuscitation 1992;23:227–34.

53. Mutschler M, Nienaber U, Munzberg M, et al. The Shock Index revisited - a fast guide to transfusion requirement? A retrospective analysis on 21,853 patients derived from the TraumaRegister DGU. Crit Care 2013;17:R172.

54. Zarzaur BL, Croce MA, Fischer PE, et al. New vitals after injury: shock index for the young and age x shock index for the old. J Surg Res 2008;147:229–36.

55. Rady MY. The role of central venous oximetry, lactic acid concentration and shock index in the evaluation of clinical shock: a review. Resuscitation 1992; 24:55–60.

56. Rady MY, Rivers EP, Nowak RM. Resuscitation of the critically ill in the ED: responses of blood pressure, heart rate, shock index, central venous oxygen saturation, and lactate. Am J Emerg Med 1996;14:218–25.

57. Birkhahn RH, Gaeta TJ, Terry D, et al. Shock index in diagnosing early acute hypovolemia. Am J Emerg Med 2005;23:323–6.

58. Cannon CM, Braxton CC, Kling-Smith M, et al. Utility of the shock index in predicting mortality in traumatically injured patients. J Trauma 2009;67:1426–30.

59. Vassallo J, Horne S, Ball S, et al. Usefulness of the shock index as a secondary triage tool. J R Army Med Corps 2014. http://dx.doi.org/10.1136/jramc-2013-000178.

60. Apodaca A, Morrison J, Spott M, et al. Improvements in the hemodynamic stability of combat casualties during en-route care. Shock 2013;40:5–10.

61. Holcomb JB, Niles SE, Miller CC, et al. Prehospital physiologic data and life-saving interventions in trauma patients. Mil Med 2005;170:7–13.

62. Holcomb JB, Salinas J, McManus JM, et al. Manual vital signs reliably predict need for life-saving interventions in trauma patients. J Trauma 2005;59:821–8.

63. McManus J, Yershov AL, Ludwig D, et al. Radial pulse character relationships to systolic blood pressure and trauma outcomes. Prehosp Emerg Care 2005;9:423–8.

64. Cancio LC, Wade CE, West SA, et al. Prediction of mortality and of the need for massive transfusion in casualties arriving at combat support hospitals in Iraq. J Trauma 2008;64(2 Suppl):S51–5.

65. Salinas J. Monitoring trauma patients in the prehospital and hospital environments: the need for better monitors and advanced automation. Fort Belvoir, VA: DTIC; 2008.

66. Van Haren RM, Thorson CM, Valle EJ, et al. Novel prehospital monitor with injury acuity alarm to identify trauma patients who require lifesaving intervention. J Trauma Acute Care Surg 2014;76:743–9.
67. Moulton SL, Mulligan J, Grudic GZ, et al. Running on empty? The compensatory reserve index. J Trauma 2013;75:1053–9.
68. Convertino VA. Blood pressure measurement for accurate assessment of patient status in emergency medical settings. Aviat Space Environ Med 2012;83:614–9.
69. Van Sickle C, Schafer K, Mulligan J, et al. A sensitive shock index for real-time patient assessment during simulated hemorrhage. Aviat Space Environ Med 2013;84:907–12.
70. Muniz GW, Wampler DA, Manifold CA, et al. Promoting early diagnosis of hemodynamic instability during simulated hemorrhage with the use of a real-time decision-assist algorithm. J Trauma Acute Care Surg 2013;75(2 Suppl 2):S184–9.
71. Nadler R, Convertino VA, Gendler S, et al. The value of noninvasive measurement of the compensatory reserve index in monitoring and triage of patients experiencing minimal blood loss. Shock 2014;42:93–8.
72. Beilman GJ, Blondet JJ. Near-infrared spectroscopy-derived tissue oxygen saturation in battlefield injuries: a case series report. World J Emerg Surg 2009;4:25.
73. Soller BR, Zou F, Ryan KL, et al. Lightweight noninvasive trauma monitor for early indication of central hypovolemia and tissue acidosis: a review. J Trauma Acute Care Surg 2012;73(2 Suppl 1):S106–11.
74. Cohn S, Crookes B, Proctor KG. Near-infrared spectroscopy in resuscitation. J Trauma 2003;54(5):S199–202.
75. McKinley BA, Marvin RG, Cocanour CS, et al. Tissue hemoglobin O2 saturation during resuscitation of traumatic shock monitored using near infrared spectrometry. J Trauma 2000;48:637–42.
76. Crookes BA, Cohn SM, Bloch S, et al. Can near-infrared spectroscopy identify the severity of shock in trauma patients? J Trauma 2005;58:806–13.
77. Beilman GJ, Blondet JJ. Tissue oxygen saturation in battlefield injuries using near-infrared spectroscopy: a case series report. World J Emerg Surg 2009;4:25.
78. Beekley A, Martin MJ, Nelson T, et al. Continuous noninvasive tissue oximetry in the early evaluation of the combat casualty: a prospective study. J Trauma Acute Care Surg 2010;69(Suppl 1):S14–25.
79. Khasawneh M, Zielinski M, Jenkins D, et al. Low tissue oxygen saturation is associated with requirements for transfusion in the rural trauma population. World J Surg 2014;38:1892–7.
80. Bridges E, Beilman G. Occult hypoperfusion in seriously injured combat casualties pre/post MEDEVAC transport. Crit Care Med 2013;41(12 (Suppl0)):A67.
81. Guyette FX, Gomez H, Suffoletto B, et al. Prehospital dynamic tissue oxygen saturation response predicts in-hospital lifesaving interventions in trauma patients. J Trauma Acute Care Surg 2012;72:930–5.

Advances in Cerebral Monitoring for the Patient with Traumatic Brain Injury

Zakraus Mahdavi, MD, Naregnia Pierre-Louis, MD,
Thuy-Tien Ho, PA, Stephen A. Figueroa, MD,
DaiWai M. Olson, PhD, RN*

KEYWORDS

- Multimodal monitoring • Neurocritical care • Intensive care • Nursing
- Traumatic brain injury

KEY POINTS

- For patients with traumatic brain injury (TBI), the future of multimodal monitoring (MMM) has yet to be fully realized.
- The past 2 decades have witnessed significant technological advances that now make it possible to simultaneously monitor the physical, chemical, and electrical activity inside the skull.
- High temporal-resolution monitors are quickly replacing static "moment-in-time" measures; global cerebral monitoring is giving way to regional and even localized monitors.
- The elusive Holy Grail of MMM is a single integrated system that will provide clinicians with highly reliable and valid measures, which will guide decisions that lead to improve patient outcomes.

INTRODUCTION

The fully functional human brain relies on the complex interplay of physical, chemical, and electrical pathways. Injury along any one neurologic pathway may be noted as a change in neurologic function. Patients with traumatic brain injury (TBI) are at high risk for injury to one or more parts of multiple pathways. This gives rise to the concept that a comprehensive critical care TBI program is one that provides practitioners with a wide variety of tools to simultaneously monitor multiple parameters associated with neurologic function. The phrase multimodal monitoring (MMM) describes this dynamic process.

The primary TBI event triggers a wide host of chemical, electrical, and mechanical pathways that result in tissue damage and give rise to secondary brain injury. The secondary brain injury inflammatory cascade is a common pathway that includes

Department of Neurology and Neurotherapeutics, UT Southwestern Medical Center, 5323 Harry Hines Boulevard, Dallas, TX 75390, USA
* Corresponding author.
E-mail address: Daiwai.Olson@utsouthwestern.edu

Crit Care Nurs Clin N Am 27 (2015) 213–223
http://dx.doi.org/10.1016/j.cnc.2015.02.002
0899-5885/15/$ – see front matter © 2015 Elsevier Inc. All rights reserved.

ccnursing.theclinics.com

blood-brain barrier (BBB) disruption, generation of free radical oxygen species, migration of microglia and macrophages, thrombin-mediated effects, and inflammatory cytokines. An understanding of the parameters available to monitor for secondary brain injury is essential to manage patients in the neurocritical care unit (NCCU).

Following TBI, the 3 primary reasons for monitoring the brain are as follows:

1. To provide an early warning, which allows for an opportunity for intervention with treatment or additional monitoring if indicated,
2. To evaluate the impact of ongoing treatment, and
3. To prognosticate patient outcome.

Monitoring multiple parameters provides the clinician with both an early warning when the patient is deteriorating and data to evaluate the effectiveness of interventions. Finally, MMM provides prognostic data. This article serves to familiarize the readers with the most common MMM tools by dividing the discussion into the most common noninvasive and invasive types of monitoring that are currently used in the practice of caring for patients with TBI.

NONINVASIVE MONITORING

A "noninvasive" cerebral monitoring device does not require invasion of the protective barriers, including skin, skull, or dura. Although both invasive and noninvasive monitoring may require significant resources, the latter is attractive because of faster setup times and lower risk of infection. The primary modes of MMM in the NCCU, discussed in the following sections, are the neurologic examination, neuroimaging, ultrasound, near-infrared spectroscopy, and electrophysiological monitoring.

The Neurologic Examination

Despite significant technological advances in health care, the most efficient method of monitoring patients with TBI is performing a neurologic examination based on the history.[1,2] The history provides the examiner with clues to the mechanism of injury and potential complications.[3] The physical examination allows the practitioner to formulate treatment decisions and to assess the need for additional monitoring.[2] At a minimum, the examination should assess the level of consciousness, cranial nerves, motor examination, sensory level, and vital signs.[1]

Level of consciousness is dependent on the arousal and cognitive components derived from the reticular activating system and cerebral cortex and is graded by the awareness of self in relation to the environment.[4,5] Consciousness, evaluated in terms of eye opening, verbal assessment, and motor examination, may be scored using the Glasgow Coma Scale (GCS) or the Full Outline of Unresponsiveness (FOUR) score.[6,7] The GCS, which ranges from 3 to 15, was designed to measure the initial severity of TBI. A GCS less than or equal to 8 is typically used as a threshold to define the need for airway protection (intubation and mechanical ventilation).[8] The FOUR score, which ranges from 0 to 16, is similar to the GCS, but includes brainstem reflexes and respiratory pattern instead of the verbal component of the GCS.[9]

Pupillometer

A key element of the physical examination is the cranial nerve (CN) assessment. Assessing pupillary function examines components of CN-II (optic) and CN-III (oculomotor). The traditional method of pupillary examination, using a handheld flashlight to subjectively score the size, shape, and reactivity of the pupils, has limited interrater reliability.[10] The pupillometer is a handheld device that works by first measuring the initial size of the pupil, and then emitting a burst of light. When cranial nerves II and III are properly functioning, the stimulus from the light is carried along CN-II to the Edinger-Westphal nucleus and a motor stimulus is sent (CN-III) to cause the pupil to constrict. The pupillometer measures the speed at which the pupil constricts and also provides a neuro-pupillary index, which (based on a proprietary algorithm) takes into account the maximum and minimum pupil size as well as the constriction velocity.

Neuroimaging

Neuroimaging describes a broad array of techniques used to visually explore the dynamic relationship of the tissues and fluids housed within the skull. Traditional radiography, cerebral angiography, computed tomography (CT), PET, optical imaging, ultrasonography, MRI, and functional MRI all have roles evaluating cerebral pathology. This article focuses on care of the patient with TBI, so the discussion focuses on CT, MRI, and ultrasound technology.

Brain Computed Tomography

The CT scanner, a "donut-shaped" gantry housing both an x-ray source and an x-ray sensor collects data by rotating on a 360-degree axis and obtaining x-ray images from multiple angles. Computer algorithms reconstruct an axial image (slice) from these data. Brain CT is widely accepted as a standard to evaluate patients with known or suspected TBI.[11,12]

When there is a sudden decline in neurologic status, an emergent noncontrast CT scan may be obtained to evaluate for a new acute intracranial process. A noncontrasted brain CT can identify traumatic subarachnoid hemorrhage, subdural hemorrhage, epidural hemorrhage, cerebral contusion, or intraparenchymal/cerebral hemorrhage. A head CT with contrast can be obtained to assess for BBB disruption, which is seen with abscesses, tumors, or demyelination. Elevated intracranial pressure (ICP) may be suspected if the brain CT reveals cerebral edema or obstructive hydrocephalus.

MRI

Although MRI has limited utility in the acute TBI setting, it is used frequently to obtain clarification once the patient is stabilized. Acute ischemia results in a decrease in intracellular water diffusion, known as restricted diffusion, which will appear bright on diffusion-weighted imaging and dark on apparent diffusion coefficient. MRI may be useful in evaluating traumatic versus nontraumatic hemorrhage. In some cases, it may be difficult to determine if a hemorrhage is resulting from trauma or tumor. Hyperacute blood may present as isointense on unenhanced T1 images. After several hours, this blood will later appear hyperintense. To differentiate this further, location is important: hypertensive hemorrhages typically appear in the brainstem or deep basal ganglia, whereas hemorrhages secondary to primary tumors typically appear in the white matter, and hemorrhages due to metastatic disease appear in the gray-white junctions. Contrast enhancement also may provide a clue: in the setting of primary hemorrhages, it may take days to weeks to show enhancement. However, enhancement seen contiguous with the hemorrhage shortly after the ictus may suggest a related tumor. Finally, presentation of edema surrounding the hemorrhage also may signal an underlying tumor. Repeating MRI several weeks after the initial hemorrhage would be necessary to further delineate the presence of a tumor.[13]

Ultrasound

Since the development of medical ultrasound technology in the 1980s, ultrasound has played a vital role in the NCCU. Ultrasound generates high-frequency sound waves that are reflected off tissues in the body. On the ultrasound, the amount of reflected sound is noted in the image by its color. Fluids conduct sound waves better than solids, and therefore appear dark, and calcified structures (bones) appear white because more sound waves are reflected back. Air also is a strong reflector.[14] Ultrasound has been repeatedly validated in neurocritical care as an imaging technique that can be used to examine both dynamic and static structures in real time.[15]

Carotid Doppler

Carotid Doppler ultrasound is used primarily to assess for stenosis in the carotid arteries of the neck.[16] It can provide information about the amount of disease present by assessing the percentage of diameter reduction, plaque length, and the hemodynamic effects of the plaque.[17] The vertebral arteries also can be assessed during the study. Data from carotid Dopplers should be compared with data from other techniques, such as CT, MRI or MRI-angiography, and conventional angiography, to have a better understanding of the arterial stenosis.

Transcranial Doppler

Transcranial Doppler (TCD) ultrasound may provide insight into ongoing risk for secondary brain injury following TBI.[16] TCD has multiple applications, including evaluating for intracranial vascular disease, monitoring vasospasm in the setting of subarachnoid hemorrhage, detection of cerebral microemboli, and screening children with sickle cell disease.[17] Direct visualization of the brain using ultrasound can be done as well to monitor for midline shift, hydrocephalus, and hemorrhage.[18] Measurement from flow velocity tracings and calculated values (eg, Lindegaard ratio) are useful to evaluate for cerebral artery vasospasm.[17,19] The TCD Pulsatility Index may provide a noninvasive estimation of ICP by acting as a measure of increased resistance in distal arterioles.[20]

Optic Nerve Sheath Diameter

Bedside ocular ultrasound to measure the optic nerve sheath diameter (ONSD), first reported in 1964, is an emerging noninvasive technique.[21] The ONSD can be measured using standard ultrasound equipment and examined as a surrogate measure of ICP.[22–25] Two studies reported data from 42 patients and defined an abnormal ICP as greater than 20 cm H_2O (14.7 mm Hg).[22,23] Given limited available data, the utility of ONSD to provide meaningful correlates for ICP is not yet fully established.

Near-Infrared Spectroscopy

Near-infrared spectroscopy (NIRS) has been used in limited capacity to monitor regional cerebral blood flow (CBF) and cerebral oxygen levels. The ability to accurately and noninvasively monitor CBF and cerebral oxygen has long been a goal of the NCCU community, but accuracy of NIRS in TBI limits the clinical utility of this technology.[11,26] The combination of NIRS and ultrasound Doppler analysis is currently being explored as an alternative to NIRS alone to provide a more robust measure of CBF and cerebral oxygen values.[27]

Electroencephalography

Human-based electroencephalography (EEG) monitoring was developed in the middle of the 20th century. Traditionally, this was almost exclusively used for seizure detection and monitoring. Advanced signal processing and high-speed computer processors now extend the use of EEG beyond seizure monitoring. Recent guidelines provide a strong recommendation in favor of EEG monitoring for all patients with acute brain injury with either altered consciousness or unexplained mental status change.[11]

Essential Electroencephalography Monitoring

Similar to the ability of an electrocardiogram to provide an electrical view of heart activity, an EEG provides an electrical view of brain activity. The EEG waveform reflects the difference in electrical charge between 2 electrodes. If both have the same charge, the difference is 0 (flat EEG). Any difference in electrical potential between 2 electrodes appears as a change in the amplitude (height) of the EEG waveform. Monitoring for change(s) in waveform morphology has the potential to provide clinicians with a greater understanding (beyond seizure management)of neuronal activity. This information can theoretically be used to abate or reduce secondary brain injury.

Compressed Spectral Array and Density Spectral Array

Both compressed spectral array (CSA) and density spectral array (DSA) are hypothesized to have prognostic and diagnostic value in TBI.[28] The lower cost and increased availability of high-speed computing has ushered a new era of availability for these signal-processing techniques. CSA algorithms transform the raw EEG signal into a graphical display of the relationship between the frequency (horizontal axis) and amplitude (vertical axis) of the EEG signal. DSA incorporates time as a variable and displays a color-coded relationship for frequency and amplitude (vertical axis) over time (horizontal axis). CSA and DSA can be used in the NCCU to assess for sedation, monitor for the presence of seizure, and potentially prognosticate outcome after TBI.[29]

Bispectral Index Monitoring

The Bispectral Index provides high-quality temporal monitoring of signal-processed EEG (spEEG).[30] Although controversial, spEEG has effectively monitored the depth of sedation over time for neurologically injured patients.[31–33] It must be noted that spEEG monitors do not evaluate responsiveness, and should be used in conjunction with subjective sedation assessment tools to get a more comprehensive picture of the patient's sedation status.[34] Suppression-ratio from spEEG can be used to monitor patients who are in burst-suppression (eg, pentobarbital coma).[35]

INVASIVE MONITORING

For the purpose of this article, the term "invasive" is defined as passing through, or *invading*, at least one of the protective barriers of the body (eg, skin, bone, dura). As such, an invasive monitor is any device that requires invasion of one body cavity or more to provide meaningful data. For patients with TBI, invasive monitoring is primarily used to measure ICP, cerebral oxygen, CBF, and brain temperature.

Intracranial Pressure

ICP monitoring developed and evolved during the last century to become emblematic of NCCU MMM.[36] The origins of ICP monitoring can be traced to the Monro-Kellie doctrine, which summarizes the work initially published by Monro in 1783 and later confirmed in a publication by Dr Kellie in 1821.[37] This doctrine posits that, within the cranial vault, 3 contents (blood, brain/tissue, and cerebrospinal fluid [CSF]) exist in a state of equilibrium that defines the ICP.

The dynamic relationship described by the Monro-Kellie doctrine implies that ICP is equally distributed throughout the intracranial vault. This information was quickly absorbed into CSF flow diversion following the first ventricular puncture in 1881 by Wernicke.[38] The modern support for ICP monitoring is due in large part to the assumption that the Monro-Kellie doctrine accurately describes intracranial pathology and that pressure within the ventricles reflects pressure throughout the intracranial space. Recently, several investigators have questioned whether the Monro-Kellie doctrine fully accounts for intracranial dynamics.[37–39]

ICP should provide the practitioner with insight to a relative increase or decrease of one or more of these contents.[40] There are neither clinical trial data nor class I evidence to support ICP as a predictor of outcome.[41] There is, however, an association between increased ICP burden and poor outcome after TBI.[42] Studies have demonstrated that when ICP is unresponsive to medical therapy, there is an increase in poor outcome.[43–49] Recent literature has begun to question the practice variation in ICP monitoring,[50,51] and the optimal target for interventions aimed to treat ICP.[52]

Intracranial Pressure via External Ventricular Drain

The use of an external ventricular drain (EVD) to monitor ICP is generally considered to be a cornerstone of neurologic monitoring.[36] The modern technique of ICP monitoring via EVD, detailed by Tillmanns in 1908, advocated for the use of a sterile flexible hollow catheter placed through the Kocher point into one of the lateral ventricles. This is then connected to a drainage bag. Pressure can be measured through the use of a pressure transducer attached to the system. This pressure transducer not only measures intracranial pressure, but also produces a waveform that provides increased detail. Lundberg described the elements of the waveform in 1960. The waveform consists of 3 components: P1, P2, and P3. The amplitude of these waveforms varies with changes in intracranial compliance. Normally, P1 is greater than P2, which is greater than P3. With increasing ICPs, the amplitudes of all 3 components of the waveform will increase, but eventually, P2 will have a larger amplitude than P1 or P3.

Intracranial Pressure via Fiberoptic Monitoring

Fiberoptic ICP monitoring was introduced more than 3 decades ago as a means to measure ICP in the intraparenchymal space. The recognized advantages of ICP via fiberoptic or pneumatic device are based on the location of the pressure transducer. Locating the transducer at the tip of the catheter (inside the skull) eliminates the need to constantly re-level the transducer.[40] Intraparenchymal monitoring also provides a more direct measure of pressures in the lesion or in the penumbra. A variety of studies have been conducted that support the hypothesis that fiberoptic monitoring provides a reliable and similar ICP compared with EVD.[53–56] However, specific conditions exist in which the ICP measured in tissue may be significantly different (compartmentalized) from the ICP measured in the ventricle, wherein both measures would be considered reliable.[40] This is functionally similar to the construct that blood pressure measured in the aortic arch may be different from blood pressure measured in the radial artery, although both are reliable.

Cerebral Perfusion Pressure

Cerebral perfusion pressure (CPP) is a calculated value based on the patient's ICP and mean arterial blood pressure (MAP). Specifically, CPP is equal to MAP minus ICP.[40] Guidelines support CPP monitoring as an adjunctive therapy whenever ICP monitoring is deployed.[57] The Brain Trauma Foundation guidelines suggest that an optimal CPP of 50 to 60 mm Hg should be the goal in severe acute TBI. Studies examining adherence to this guideline have found that although adherence is generally low, most CPPs outside of the boundaries tend to be self-regulated hyperperfusion (CPP >70 mm Hg) and there are inadequate data to suggest that practitioners should intentionally elevate ICP or lower MAP to drive down perfusion pressures.[58]

Cerebral Oxygen Monitoring

Oxygen-rich blood is delivered anteriorly from the carotid arteries and posteriorly from the vertebrobasilar arteries.[59] The brain, which does not store oxygen, requires a continuous supply of oxygen to maintain function, which directly links CBF with cerebral oxygenation and metabolism. Systemic levels of oxygen (Pao_2 and SaO2) do not necessarily reflect brain tissue oxygen levels. Continuously monitoring brain oxygen levels can be measured in several ways via invasive and noninvasive methods. First, the partial pressure of brain tissue oxygen (PbtO2) can be measured invasively by using a fiberoptic probe placed directly into the brain parenchyma.[60] PbtO2 is a form of local cerebral oxygen monitoring because it provides a direct reflection of the oxygen pressure in a very small area of the brain surrounding the tip of the fiberoptic probe. The second form of brain oxygen monitoring is jugular venous oxygen saturation (SjO2). Continuous SjO2 monitoring is accomplished by placing a fiberoptic catheter retrograde into the internal jugular vein such that the tip of the catheter sits at the jugular venous bulb. Monitoring the SjO2 provides a reflection of global (hemispheric) oxygen reserve with a typical value between 60% and 80% venous oxygen saturation. Values less than 50% can represent ischemia, systemic hypoxia, or decreased cardiac output.

Cerebral Blood Flow Monitoring

Normal CBF is roughly 45 to 65 mL/100 g of brain tissue.[40] The use of thermal diffusion flowmetry (TDF) provides an invasive measure of CBF in a highly focalized region of the brain. The ultimate goal of CBF monitoring is to provide the clinician with assurance of preserved adequate CBF or to provide data that would trigger a treatment change. There are no randomized clinical trials associating CBF monitoring in TBI with improved patient outcomes.[11] Therefore, invasive CBF monitoring is considered to provide primarily prognostic, diagnostic, and research-related data. However, recent guidelines support the use of TDF to aid in the detection of ischemia after subarachnoid hemorrhage and to identify focal ischemia or infarct (confined to the area in which the CBF probe is placed).[11]

Brain Temperature Monitoring

Human tissues survive only across a relatively narrow temperature range of roughly 31 to 41°C. In concert with advances in therapeutic temperature management, continuous temperature monitoring has grown in popularity, is relatively inexpensive, and readily integrates with most existing bedside monitors. The vast majority of continuous temperature monitoring relies on indwelling urinary catheters, rectal probes, or esophageal probes.[61] However, invasive brain temperature monitoring has been added as a feature to several other invasive monitoring devices (eg, PbtO2 or CBF). Relatively few studies have examined the impact of brain temperature monitoring in clinical trials. The difference between brain temperature and core body temperature may be associated with changes in cerebral perfusion.[62–64]

SUMMARY

For patients with TBI, the future of MMM has yet to be fully realized. The past 2 decades have witnessed significant technological advances that now make it possible to simultaneously monitor the physical, chemical, and electrical activity inside the skull. High temporal-resolution monitors are quickly replacing static "moment-in-time" measures. Global cerebral monitoring is giving way to regional and even localized monitors.[65] The elusive Holy Grail of MMM is a single integrated system that will provide clinicians with highly reliable and valid measures that will guide decisions that lead to improved patient outcomes.

REFERENCES

1. American Association of Neuroscience Nurses. AANN core curriculum for neuroscience nursing. 5th edition. Glenview (IL): American Association of Neuroscience Nurses; 2010.
2. Singhal NS, Josephson SA. A practical approach to neurologic evaluation in the intensive care unit. J Crit Care 2014;29(4):627–33.
3. Olson D, Meek L, Lynch J. Accurate patient history contributes to differentiating diabetes insipidus: a case study. J Neurosci Nurs 2004;36(4):228–30.
4. Plum F, Posner JB. The diagnosis of stupor and coma. 3rd edition. Philadelphia: Davis; 1980.
5. Mazzoni P, Pearson TS, Rowland LP, et al. Merritt's neurology handbook. Philadelphia: Lippincott Williams & Wilkins; 2006.
6. Teasdale G, Jennett B. Assessment of coma and impaired consciousness. A practical scale. Lancet 1974;2(7872):81–4.
7. Wijdicks EF, Bamlet WR, Maramattom BV, et al. Validation of a new coma scale: the FOUR score. Ann Neurol 2005;58(4):585–93.
8. Kesinger MR, Nagy LR, Sequeira DJ, et al. A standardized trauma care protocol decreased in-hospital mortality of patients with severe traumatic brain injury at a teaching hospital in a middle-income country. Injury 2014;45(9):1350–4.
9. Iyer VN, Mandrekar JN, Danielson RD, et al. Validity of the FOUR score coma scale in the medical intensive care unit. Mayo Clin Proc 2009;84(8):694–701.
10. Meeker M, Du R, Bacchetti P, et al. Pupil examination: validity and clinical utility of an automated pupillometer. J Neurosci Nurs 2005;37(1):34–40.
11. Le Roux P, Menon DK, Citerio G, et al. Consensus summary statement of the international multidisciplinary consensus conference on multimodality monitoring in neurocritical care: a statement for healthcare professionals from the neurocritical care society and the European Society of Intensive Care Medicine. Neurocrit Care 2014. PMID: 25208678 [Epub ahead of print].
12. Vespa PM. Imaging and decision-making in neurocritical care. Neurol Clin 2014; 32(1):211–24.
13. Carhuapoma JR, Mayer SA, Hanley DF. Intracerebral hemorrhage. Cambridge (United Kingdom); New York: Cambridge University Press; 2010.
14. Abu-Zidan FM, Hefny AF, Corr P. Clinical ultrasound physics. J Emerg Trauma Shock 2011;4(4):501–3.
15. Bilotta F, Dei Giudici L, Lam A, et al. Ultrasound-based imaging in neurocritical care patients: a review of clinical applications. Neurol Res 2013;35(2):149–58.
16. Bouzat P, Oddo M, Payen JF. Transcranial Doppler after traumatic brain injury: is there a role? Curr Opin Crit Care 2014;20(2):153–60.
17. Katz ML, Alexandrov AV. A practical guide to transcranial Doppler examinations. 1st edition. Littleton, CO: Summer Pub; 2003.
18. Caricato A, Pitoni S, Montini L, et al. Echography in brain imaging in intensive care unit: state of the art. World J Radiol 2014;6(9):636–42.
19. Rigamonti A, Ackery A, Baker AJ. Transcranial Doppler monitoring in subarachnoid hemorrhage: a critical tool in critical care. Can J Anaesth 2008;55(2):112–23.

20. Manno EM. Transcranial Doppler ultrasonography in the neurocritical care unit. Crit Care Clin 1997;13(1):79–104.

21. Hayreh SS. Pathogenesis of oedema of the optic disc (papiloedema); a preliminary report. Br J Ophthalmol 1964;48:522–43.

22. Lashutka MK, Chandra A, Murray HN, et al. The relationship of intraocular pressure to intracranial pressure. Ann Emerg Med 2004;43(5):585–91.

23. Kimberly HH, Shah S, Marill K, et al. Correlation of optic nerve sheath diameter with direct measurement of intracranial pressure. Acad Emerg Med 2008;15(2):201–4.

24. Cammarata G, Ristagno G, Cammarata A, et al. Ocular ultrasound to detect intracranial hypertension in trauma patients. J Trauma 2011;71(3):779–81.

25. Major R, Girling S, Boyle A. Ultrasound measurement of optic nerve sheath diameter in patients with a clinical suspicion of raised intracranial pressure. Emerg Med J 2011;28(8):679–81.

26. Schneider A, Minnich B, Hofstatter E, et al. Comparison of four near-infrared spectroscopy devices shows that they are only suitable for monitoring cerebral oxygenation trends in preterm infants. Acta Paediatr 2014;103(9):934–8.

27. Schytz HW, Guo S, Jensen LT, et al. A new technology for detecting cerebral blood flow: a comparative study of ultrasound tagged NIRS and 133Xe-SPECT. Neurocrit Care 2012;17(1):139–45.

28. Goldfine AM, Victor JD, Conte MM, et al. Determination of awareness in patients with severe brain injury using EEG power spectral analysis. Clin Neurophysiol 2011;122(11):2157–68.

29. Stewart CP, Otsubo H, Ochi A, et al. Seizure identification in the ICU using quantitative EEG displays. Neurology 2010;75(17):1501–8.

30. Olson DM, Thoyre SM, Peterson ED, et al. A randomized evaluation of bispectral index-augmented sedation assessment in neurological patients. Neurocrit Care 2009;11(1):20–7.

31. James ML, Olson DM, Graffagnino C. A pilot study of cerebral and haemodynamic physiological changes during sedation with dexmedetomidine or propofol in patients with acute brain injury. Anaesth Intensive Care 2012;40(6):949–57.

32. Olson DM. Combining observational and physiologic sedation assessment tools [Dissertation]. Chapel Hill (NC): Nursing, The University of North Carolina; 2007.

33. Olson DM, Zomorodi MG, James ML, et al. Exploring the impact of augmenting sedation assessment with physiologic monitors. Aust Crit Care 2014;27:145–50.

34. Arbour R, Waterhouse J, Seckel MA, et al. Correlation between the sedation-agitation scale and the bispectral index in ventilated patients in the intensive care unit. Heart Lung 2009;38(4):336–45.

35. Arbour RB. Continuous nervous system monitoring, EEG, the bispectral index, and neuromuscular transmission. AACN Clin Issues 2003;14(2):185–207.

36. Srinivasan VM, O'Neill BR, Jho D, et al. The history of external ventricular drainage. J Neurosurg 2013;120:228–36.

37. Macintyre I. A hotbed of medical innovation: George Kellie (1770-1829), his colleagues at Leith and the Monro-Kellie doctrine. J Med Biogr 2013;22(2):93–100.

38. Mascarenhas S, Vilela GH, Carlotti C, et al. The new ICP minimally invasive method shows that the Monro-Kellie doctrine is not valid. Acta Neurochir Suppl 2012;114:117–20.

39. Sahuquillo J, Poca MA, Arribas M, et al. Interhemispheric supratentorial intracranial pressure gradients in head-injured patients: are they clinically important? J Neurosurg 1999;90(1):16–26.

40. Hickey JV, Olson DM. Intracranial hypertension: theory and management of increased intracranial pressure. In: Hickey JV, editor. The clinical practice of

neurological and neurosurgical nursing. 6th edition. Philadelphia: Wolters Kluwer/ Lippincott Williams & Wilkins Health; 2009. p. 270–307.

41. Czosnyka M, Pickard JD. Monitoring and interpretation of intracranial pressure. J Neurol Neurosurg Psychiatry 2004;75(6):813–21.

42. Kaye AH, Brownbill D. Postoperative intracranial pressure in patients operated on for cerebral aneurysms following subarachnoid hemorrhage. J Neurosurg 1981; 54(6):726–32.

43. Bailes JE, Spetzler RF, Hadley MN, et al. Management morbidity and mortality of poor-grade aneurysm patients. J Neurosurg 1990;72(4):559–66.

44. Citerio G, Gaini SM, Tomei G, et al. Management of 350 aneurysmal subarachnoid hemorrhages in 22 Italian neurosurgical centers. Intensive Care Med 2007;33(9):1580–6.

45. Hase U, Reulen HJ, Fenske A, et al. Intracranial pressure and pressure volume relation in patients with subarachnoid haemorrhage (SAH). Acta Neurochir 1978;44(1–2):69–80.

46. Hayashi M, Marukawa S, Fujii H, et al. Intracranial pressure in patients with diffuse cerebral arterial spasm following ruptured intracranial aneurysms. Acta Neurochir 1978;44(1–2):81–95.

47. Heuer GG, Smith MJ, Elliott JP, et al. Relationship between intracranial pressure and other clinical variables in patients with aneurysmal subarachnoid hemorrhage. J Neurosurg 2004;101(3):408–16.

48. Soehle M, Chatfield DA, Czosnyka M, et al. Predictive value of initial clinical status, intracranial pressure and transcranial Doppler pulsatility after subarachnoid haemorrhage. Acta Neurochir 2007;149(6):575–83.

49. Meixensberger J, Vath A, Jaeger M, et al. Monitoring of brain tissue oxygenation following severe subarachnoid hemorrhage. Neurol Res 2003;25(5):445–50.

50. Olson DM, Batjer HH, Abdulkadir K, et al. Measuring and monitoring ICP in neurocritical care: results from a national practice survey. Neurocrit Care 2014;20(1):15–20.

51. Olson DM, Lewis LS, Bader MK, et al. Significant practice pattern variations associated with intracranial pressure monitoring. J Neurosci Nurs 2013;45(4):186–93.

52. Chesnut R. Intracranial pressure monitoring: headstone or a new head start. The BEST TRIP trial in perspective. Intensive Care Med 2013;39:1–4.

53. Gopinath SP, Robertson CS, Contant CF, et al. Clinical evaluation of a miniature strain-gauge transducer for monitoring intracranial pressure. Neurosurgery 1995;36(6):1137–40 [discussion: 1140–1].

54. Eide PK, Holm S, Sorteberg W. Simultaneous monitoring of static and dynamic intracranial pressure parameters from two separate sensors in patients with cerebral bleeds: comparison of findings. Biomed Eng Online 2012;11:66.

55. Chambers IR, Banister K, Mendelow AD. Intracranial pressure within a developing intracerebral haemorrhage. Br J Neurosurg 2001;15(2):140–1.

56. Koskinen LO, Olivecrona M. Clinical experience with the intraparenchymal intracranial pressure monitoring Codman MicroSensor system. Neurosurgery 2005; 56(4):693–8 [discussion: 693–8].

57. Helbok R, Olson DM, Le Roux PD, et al. Intracranial pressure and cerebral perfusion pressure monitoring in non-TBI patients: special considerations. Neurocrit Care 2014. PMID: 25208677 [Epub ahead of print].

58. Griesdale DE, Ortenwall V, Norena M, et al. Adherence to guidelines for management of cerebral perfusion pressure and outcome in patients who have severe traumatic brain injury. J Crit Care 2014;30:111–5.

59. Blumenfeld H. Neuroanatomy through clinical cases. Sunderland (MA): Sinauer; 2002.

60. Littlejohns LR, Bader MK, March K. Brain tissue oxygen monitoring in severe brain injury, I. research and usefulness in critical care. Crit Care Nurse 2003; 23(4):17–25 [quiz: 26–7].
61. Olson DM, Grissom JL, Dombrowski K. The evidence base for nursing care and monitoring of patients during therapeutic temperature management. Ther Hypothermia Temp Manag 2011;1(4):209–17.
62. Suehiro E, Fujisawa H, Koizumi H, et al. Significance of differences between brain temperature and core temperature (delta T) during mild hypothermia in patients with diffuse axonal injury. Neurol Med Chir (Tokyo) 2011;51(8):551–5.
63. Gupta AK, Al-Rawi PG, Hutchinson PJ, et al. Effect of hypothermia on brain tissue oxygenation in patients with severe head injury. Br J Anaesth 2002;88(2):188–92.
64. Poli S, Purrucker J, Priglinger M, et al. Induction of cooling with a passive head and neck cooling device: effects on brain temperature after stroke. Stroke 2013;44(3):708–13.
65. Olson DM. Multimodal neurological monitoring. In: Kaplow R, Hardin SR, editors. Critical care nursing: synergy for optimal outcomes. Sudbury (MA): Jones and Bartlett; 2007. p. 359–74.

Considerations for Neuroprotection in the Traumatic Brain Injury Population

CrossMark

Karen S. Bergman, PhD, RN, CNRN[a],*, Valerie Beekmans, RN, BSN[b], Jeff Stromswold, RN, BSN, CCRN[b]

KEYWORDS

- Trauma • Brain injury • Neuroprotection • Cooling • Craniectomy

KEY POINTS

- The brain undergoes complex pathophysiologic changes following a traumatic injury, and efforts should be made to decrease the amount of secondary injury.
- There is evidence to support the use of cooling, craniectomy, and medications as neuroprotective measures to save the brain following traumatic injury.
- Cooling for all persons with severe traumatic brain injury is not supported in the evidence; however, cooling may be beneficial to reduce intracranial pressure.
- Craniectomy may be beneficial in the management of increased intracranial pressure; however, current research does not support improved outcomes for patients, and further research is needed.
- Severe traumatic brain injury is associated with a high rate of death or disability; nurses are key in monitoring and treating secondary brain injury in efforts to save the brain.
- Further research is needed to improve knowledge of neuroprotection following traumatic brain injury.

INTRODUCTION

Traumatic brain injury (TBI) is a contributing factor in approximately 30% of all injury-related deaths in the United States.[1] The Centers for Disease Control and Prevention estimated the direct and indirect cost of TBI in 2010 to be $76.5 billion, with the medical care for those with severe TBI accounting for 90% of those costs. Approximately 5.3 million Americans are living with a disability as a result of TBI, affecting all aspects of their life and their ability to function as contributing members of society.[1]

Disclosures: The authors have nothing to disclose and no conflicts of interest.
a Western Michigan University/Bronson Methodist Hospital, 601 John Street, Box 88, Kalamazoo, MI 49008, USA; b Neuro Critical Care, Bronson Methodist Hospital, 601 John Street, Box 88, Kalamazoo, MI 49007, USA
* Corresponding author.
E-mail address: bergmank@bronsonhg.org

Crit Care Nurs Clin N Am 27 (2015) 225–233
http://dx.doi.org/10.1016/j.cnc.2015.02.009
0899-5885/15/$ – see front matter © 2015 Elsevier Inc. All rights reserved.

TBI damages the neurons of the brain in both direct and indirect ways. Direct damage is caused by the initial injury compressing, twisting, or otherwise damaging the neuron, resulting in neuronal dysfunction or neuronal death. The aims of medical and nursing therapies for management of brain injury are to limit the effects of secondary brain injury, which is caused by a myriad of cellular and pathophysiologic mechanisms. Secondary injury is triggered by the initial injury and then leads to further brain damage as a result of altered cerebral blood flow, altered cerebrovascular autoregulation, changes in cerebral metabolism, and low cerebral oxygenation. Further damage to neurons can occur by excessive release of glutamate, an excitatory neurotransmitter, and the influx of calcium and sodium into the intracellular space.[2] Minimizing the effects of the secondary injury to the brain following the initial injury is the focus of nursing care in the days to weeks following the trauma.

Neuroprotection is a concept that health care providers use to optimize treatments in such a way that the neuronal damage or loss is minimized, and patient outcomes are improved. This article summarizes areas in which research has previously supported or refuted the brain-protecting efforts of procedures or medications.

COOLING

Therapeutic hypothermia has been studied for more than a decade as a neuroprotective strategy for patients after cardiac arrest.[3] The 2011 National Institute for Health and Clinical Excellence guidelines support the use of hypothermia to 32°C to 34°C for 12 to 24 hours following cardiac arrest with slow rewarming to improve neurologic outcome for comatose patients with return of spontaneous circulation.[4]

The pathophysiology of cooling as a neuroprotective mechanism is complex and involves a multitude of responses at the cellular level to the ischemia or injury. This article provide an overview of the pathophysiology in order for nurses to better understand the background of why cooling brain-injured patients may or may not be beneficial. Ischemia or injury to the brain causes the release of excitatory amino acids and glutamate. Neuronal exposure to the excess levels of these substances causes inflammation, edema, and accelerated cell death. In addition, ischemia or injury to the neuron causes a deficit in the oxygen, ATP, and glucose needed for normal cellular function. Hypothermia is able to decrease cerebral metabolic rate as well as reduce the inflammatory response, thus protecting the brain by decreasing the secondary injury.[5,6]

With the promising trials supporting the use of therapeutic hypothermia for the postarrest population, it became an area of interest to determine whether the TBI population would also have improved outcomes with the use of cooling. Several factors come into play when assessing the quality of studies supporting or refuting the effects of therapeutic hypothermia in the brain-injured population, such as when to cool (prophylactic vs targeted management if intracranial pressure [ICP] is increased), what methods to use to cool (superficial vs intravascular), how long to cool, what temperature is best, how to rewarm, and which combinations of these factors produce the best outcomes. This article uses the therapeutic moderate hypothermia range of 32°C to 35°C, because most studies are within this range.

Two large multicenter trials were conducted to determine the effect on early hypothermia after severe brain injury, targeting overall hypothermia as a neuroprotectant and not as a treatment of ICP. These trials were the North American Brain Injury Study: Hypothermia I and II.[7,8] Patients were randomized to cooling to 35°C, 33°C, or normothermia with standard of care for severe TBI. Patients were cooled quickly (<6 hours to target temperatures); however, no significant improvement in neurologic outcome or mortality was seen in either trial.

Meta-analysis is a means to aggregate data from several similarly designed studies in order to analyze the larger set of data. Three meta-analyses on the role of therapeutic hypothermia show mixed results. The earliest study reviewed was by Harris and colleagues[9] in 2002, and they analyzed 7 randomized controlled trials (RCTs) and found hypothermia to not be beneficial for the outcomes of ICP or Glasgow Outcomes Score ($P = .2$ and $P = .3$ respectively). Li and Yang[10] conducted a meta-analysis of 13 studies investigating moderate hypothermia versus normothermia and found a nonsignificant 21% improvement in neurologic outcome in the hypothermia group ($P = .12$). Crossley and colleagues[11] combined data from 18 trials and were able to find a significant reduction in mortality and reduction in poor outcome in the hypothermia groups. These meta-analyses cite heterogeneity (or differences among the persons in the studies) as a possible cause of the mixed results of trials on hypothermia for severe TBI.

The Brain Trauma Foundation publishes guidelines on the management of severe TBI, which can be located at braintrauma.org. Their findings are that there is insufficient evidence to support a level I or II recommendation, and that there is insufficient evidence to support the routine use of hypothermia for all patients with severe TBI. However, in the aggregate data from several studies, there was a decrease in mortality risk when temperatures were maintained hypothermic for greater than 48 hours.[12]

Hypothermia for the purpose of controlling ICP may have more promise than overall hypothermia to improve neurologic outcome. The Eurotherm3235 Trial[13] is an ongoing RCT including more than 12 countries to investigate cooling to a temperature of 32°C to 35° to reduce ICP. Pilot data published in 2013[14] show good feasibility of the protocol in getting patients into the study and reaching target temperatures within 4 hours and maintaining that target for at least 48 hours. Full study results are pending. Sadaka and Veremakis[15] published a systematic review of 18 studies involving hypothermia for ICP control. In all studies, routine care for ICP greater than 20 mm Hg included sedatives, narcotics, neuromuscular blockers if needed, and hyperosmolar therapy. Neurosurgery was done when lesions required evacuation. Thirteen of these studies were RCTs comparing therapeutic hypothermia with normothermia with the outcome of ICP, and in all studies there were significant differences in reduction of ICP for the hypothermia groups. These studies support that, after basic management of ICP has been initiated, a secondary approach of therapeutic hypothermia may be beneficial for reduction of ICP.

In summary, routine cooling of patients with severe TBI is not sufficiently supported in the literature at this time. Therapeutic hypothermia may be beneficial for the management of ICP that is refractory to initial therapies such as sedation and hyperosmolar therapy.

CRANIECTOMY

Decompressive craniectomy (DC) is a neurosurgical procedure used to relieve intracranial hypertension in brain-injured patients. DC is typically reserved for persons who have increased ICP that is refractory to medical management. When medical care (positioning, pharmacologic approaches, cooling) ceases to control ICP (sustained increases in ICP >20 mm Hg), removing a large portion of the skull on 1 or both sides, along with opening of the dura, allows the cerebral edema to expand outside the limits of the cranial vault.[16,17] Allowing the brain to swell outside of the normally enclosed cranial vault prevents cerebral herniation and should reduce ICP and improve cerebral blood flow.[18] A meta-analysis of the outcomes of ICP and cerebral perfusion pressure (CPP) following DC found that DC effectively decreases ICP and increases CPP in persons with refractory increases of ICP.[19]

An RCT published by Cooper and colleagues[20] (2011) compared outcomes at 6 months between persons after early bifrontotemporoparietal DC and standard care for management of intracranial hypertension. They randomized 155 adults with severe TBI, and those with craniectomy had better controlled ICP and fewer days in the intensive care unit; however, there was an equal rate of death between groups, and at 6 months the odds for having a worse outcome on the Glasgow Outcomes Score–Extended were worse for the craniectomy group (odds ratio, 1.84; $P = .03$). Despite the unpromising results of this study, clinicians continue to use DC as a method to treat refractory intracranial hypertension. There may be other factors to consider, such as bilateral versus unilateral craniectomy, timing of craniectomy, and differences in patient characteristics, that may not have been reflected in this trail.

With regard to timing of DC, most clinicians agree that craniectomy should be performed as a secondary approach, meaning that the patient has failed conservative methods to decrease or control ICP. Nirula and colleagues[21] (2014) evaluated DC performed as a primary treatment versus as a secondary therapy, assessing the timing of the DC. Their findings for 264 patients who received craniectomies showed no survival benefit with early primary DC (relative risk, 1.07; $P = .77$). Chibbaro and colleagues[22] (2011) studied 147 patients with severe TBI and found younger age and earlier DC (within 9 hours from trauma) to have a significant effect on Glasgow Outcomes Score ($P<.0001$ and $P<.03$ respectively). As can be seen from these two studies, there is still no optimal prescribed timing for performing DC for any patient.

Aside from improving the ICP and CPP of persons with refractory intracranial hypertension, there should be some long-term benefit of performing the DC, otherwise the risks may outweigh the benefits. Known risks for DC include herniation of the brain outside the skull, subdural effusion, hydrocephalus, and infection,[23] thus the surgery should be warranted in order to subject a patient to such risks. Ahmadi and colleagues[24] (2010) performed an outcome analysis of 131 patients with severe TBI who underwent DC. Among their sample, 48% died in the hospital, 20% were discharged in a vegetative state, 24% had severe disability, and 7% had moderate disability. Thirty patients with Glasgow Outcomes Score greater than 2 gave detailed outcome information, including presence of depression, neurologic deficits, and cognitive test performances. Even though the patients had a great deal of disability, patient-reported abilities at activities of daily living and quality of life were not deemed to be poor. This raises an ethical dilemma for health care workers: even with moderate disability, the patients did not seem disappointed with their quality of life, so perhaps current measures of disability do not reflect the patients' perceptions of their disabilities in day-to-day life.

Honeybul and colleagues[25] (2013) performed a study on the longer term outcomes of patients with severe TBI who had DC and who were deemed to be severely disabled 18 months after the DC. To clarify, they only assessed the population of persons with short-term poor outcomes and not those who had better short-term outcomes. Among 20 patients, 5 remained in a vegetative state 3 years after injury, and the remaining 15 remained severely disabled after 5 years. They found that, despite the severe disability that remained after 18 months, patients may recalibrate their expectations regarding what is an acceptable quality of life. This finding again shows that what is an acceptable quality of life to people without TBI and those who survive their TBI may change over time.

Once the skull is removed for craniectomy, there needs to be a plan for replacing it, which is called cranioplasty. There is little evidence for best practice regarding cranioplasty.[26] Studies that have been published are small and find no statistically significant evidence to show the techniques that are best practice.[26,27] When the craniectomy is initially performed, the bone flap may be stored in a tissue bank or in the abdominal subcutaneous fat, per the surgeon's preference. Complication rates between these storage differences did not differ significantly in a study by Basheer and colleagues.[26] However, patients with the bone flap stored in the abdominal subcutaneous tissue had more blood loss and longer operations. The current evidence summarized by Tasiou and colleagues,[27] supports early cranioplasty to improve cerebral spinal fluid dynamics and cerebral metabolism. However, the strength of the evidence to support the timing of cranioplasty is insufficient to make a clear statement about optimal timing, thus well-designed randomized trials are needed to draw conclusions on the timing of replacing bone flaps.

In summary, DC is often used as a second-tier therapy for the management of refractory intracranial hypertension; however, the exact best practice for this surgical approach is not yet fully understood in terms of timing, 1-sided versus 2-sided removal of skull, and length of time to replace the bone via cranioplasty. It is hoped that future large-scale research trials will provide insight into this practice in order to improve outcomes of persons with severe TBI.

NEUROPROTECTION: MEDICATIONS

Although there is an increased understanding of brain injury at the cellular level, there is still a gap in the science with regard to preventing the secondary neuronal injury. Research that seems promising in animal models sometimes does not translate to a positive effect in humans, and when the medications are studied in humans there are concerns over optimal dosing and timing to provide the best outcomes.

Medications Not Supported by Research

Magnesium

Magnesium sulfate has been used for prevention of eclamptic seizures in pregnant patients with preeclampsia as well as for preventing preeclampsia escalating to eclampsia.[28] The exact mechanism of the seemingly protective effects of magnesium in pregnant patients is not fully understood but it is suggested that magnesium causes some cerebral vasodilation and thus may prevent cerebral ischemia.[29] Despite the benefits of magnesium sulfate in pregnant patients, RCT use of magnesium for neuroprotection in brain injury did not prove successful. In the Temkin and colleagues[30] (2007) RCT, patients in the magnesium groups, at both high and low doses, had worse outcomes than patients in the control group, thus not supporting the use of magnesium sulfate as a neuroprotective agent for TBI.

Corticosteroids

The goal of studies that examined corticosteroid use in brain injury was to limit lipid peroxidation, which is a harmful cause of secondary damage to neurons, as shown in animal models. The use of high-dose corticosteroids was once thought to be an option for decreasing death and disability for persons with TBI, despite the known side effects of infection risk and gastrointestinal bleeding. The CRASH trial[31] (Corticosteroid Randomisation after Significant Head Injury [CRASH] Trial Management Group) was an RCT with a 48-hour infusion of high-dose corticosteroid compared with placebo. The results showed increased mortality in the treatment versus placebo groups, thus not supporting the use of methylprednisolone with TBI. In addition,

Alderson and Roberts[32] (2009) conducted a meta-analysis of studies conducted to investigate corticosteroids and brain injury, and found that there was no improved mortality in the treatment groups and that the risk for infection and gastrointestinal bleeding was higher in the treatment groups, again not supporting use in humans.

Medications with Potential for Neuroprotection

Progesterone

In the Progesterone for the Treatment of Traumatic Brain Injury (ProTECT) study, Wright and colleagues[33] completed a randomized placebo-controlled clinical trial with 100 persons randomly assigned 4:1 to receive intravenous progesterone or placebo. Patients included in this study were adults who had Glasgow Coma Scale scores of 4 to 12, and thus were in the moderate to severe categories of brain injury. Dosing of progesterone was as follows: loading dose of 0.71 mg/kg at 14 mL/h for the first hour, then reduced to 10 mL/h (0.5 mg/kg) for 11 hours, then 10 mL/h for the total of 3 days of treatment. Seventy-seven patients received progesterone and 23 received placebo. For outcomes, there was no difference between groups for mean ICP, and severely injured persons in the progesterone group were in comas longer than the control group; however, more persons survived in the progesterone group, which likely explains this result. There was not a statistical difference in duration of posttraumatic amnesia. Thirty-day Glasgow Outcomes Score–Extended and Disability Rating Scale were used for the longer term outcomes. Persons in the progesterone group had lower 30-day mortality than controls, and for those with moderate injury the progesterone group was more likely to have moderate to good outcomes compared with the placebo group.

Xiao and colleagues[34] (2008) studied persons with severe TBI in China and included 159 persons randomized to progesterone (N = 82), or placebo (N = 77). Patients had to be within 8 hours of their injury, and were given 1.0 mg/kg of intramuscular (IM) progesterone followed by IM injections every 12 hours for 5 days. Patients in the progesterone group had more favorable Glasgow Outcomes Scores at 3 months compared with the placebo group (47% vs 31%; P = .034). Similar results held true at 6 months after injury (58% vs 42% favorable outcome; P = .048). Mortality was better for patients in the progesterone group (18%) versus the placebo group (32%) at 6 months after injury (P = .039). There were no significant differences in ICP or group differences in Glasgow Coma Score improvements in the study.

Further studies are needed to support the use of progesterone for all patients with moderate or severe TBI. ProTECT III is an ongoing study of IV progesterone within 4 hours of injury given for 96 hours for moderate to severe TBI. The Glasgow Outcomes Score–Extended is the outcome for this study. The Study of the Neuroprotective Activity of Progesterone in Severe Traumatic Brain Injury (SyNAPSe) study is a large international phase III clinical trial comparing progesterone with placebo. This study is investigating severe TBI only, with a 5-day infusion of progesterone, and the main outcome variable of Glasgow Outcomes Score. At this point, progesterone as a neuroprotective agent for TBI holds promise; however, until the larger trials are complete, the patients who should receive the medication, the optimal dosing, and the ideal time to give the medication remain unclear.

Glutamate scavengers

Glutamate is a nonessential amino acid and an excitatory neurotransmitter in the central nervous system.[35] Glutamate is necessary for normal cell function; however, increased levels can have a negative effect. Following TBI, there is an increase of glutamate in the brain's extracellular fluid that can lead to cellular edema, apoptosis, and neuronal death. Zlotnik and colleagues[36] (2012) were able to show the neuroprotective qualities of the use of glutamate scavengers, oxaloacetate, and pyruvate in animal models, with the outcomes of reduction in the loss of neurons in the hippocampus and improved neurologic outcomes in rats. Further studies are needed in animal and eventually human models to be able to consider glutamate scavengers or other methods of controlling glutamate levels (eg, hemodialysis) as a neuroprotective strategy for TBI.

Stem cell therapy

Stem cell therapy for the treatment of brain injury would allow clinicians to shift the focus from neuroprotection to neurorestoration, with the potential to restore function to people with brain injury. Although there is extensive stem cell research being performed in laboratory settings, translation of that research to humans has been slow and complex. Much of the work being done is to support the growing population of persons with neurodegenerative diseases, such as multiple sclerosis and Parkinson disease, as well as persons with stroke.[37,38] Although it is beyond the scope of this article to fully explain the intricacies of stem cell therapy, we hope to bringing this science to the attention of nurses to increase awareness that, in time, new therapies will be developed for patients with TBI.

SUMMARY

Nurses are essential for monitoring for and treating secondary brain injury. Despite decades of research on neuroprotective methods for managing severe brain injury, further studies are needed. Most likely, research will find that several therapies combined will provide the optimal neuroprotection; however, to date there is no scientifically supported combination of nursing, medical, and surgical therapies. Therapies such as cooling, craniectomy, and neuroprotective medications may need to be studied together to best understand the complexity of TBI and how to improve patient outcomes, reducing mortality and disability.

REFERENCES

1. Centers for Disease Control. Injury prevention and control: traumatic brain injury. 2014. Available at: http://www.cdc.gov/TraumaticBrainInjury/. Accessed January 15, 2015.
2. Werner C, Engelhard K. Pathophysiology of traumatic brain injury. Br J Anaesth 2007;99(1):4–9.
3. Nolan J, Morley P, Vanden Hoek T, et al. Therapeutic hypothermia after cardiac arrest. Circulation 2003;108:118–21.
4. National Institute for Health and Clinical Excellence. Therapeutic hypothermia following cardiac arrest. 2011. Available at: www.nice.org.uk. Accessed January 15, 2015.
5. Karnatovskaia L, Wartenberg K, Freeman W. Therapeutic hypothermia for neuroprotection: history, mechanisms, risks, and clinical applications. Neurohospitalist 2014;4(3):153–63.
6. Wang H, Wang B, Normoyle K, et al. Brain temperature and its fundamental properties: a review for clinical neuroscientists. Front Neurosci 2014;8:1–17.
7. Clifton G, Drever P, Valadka A, et al. Multicenter trial of early hypothermia in severe brain injury. J Neurotrauma 2009;26:393–7.
8. Clifton G, Valadka A, Zygun D, et al. Very early hypothermia induction in patients with severe brain injury (the National Acute Brain Injury Study: Hypothermia II): a randomized trial. Lancet Neurol 2011;10(2):131–9.

9. Harris O, Colford J, Good M, et al. The role of hypothermia in the management of severe brain injury: a meta-analysis. Arch Neurol 2002;59(7):1077–83.

10. Li P, Yang C. Moderate hypothermia treatment in adult patients with severe traumatic brain injury: a meta-analysis. Brain Inj 2014;28(8):1036–41.

11. Crossley S, Reid J, McLatchie R, et al. A systematic review of therapeutic hypothermia for adult patients following traumatic brain injury. Crit Care 2014; 18:R75.

12. Brain Trauma Foundation. Guidelines for the management of severe traumatic brain injury. 2007. Available at: braintrauma.org. Accessed February 1, 2015.

13. Andrews P, Sinclair H, Battison C, et al. European Society of Intensive Care Medicine study of therapeutic hypothermia for intracranial pressure reduction after traumatic brain injury (the Eurotherm3235Trial). Trials 2011;12(8):1–12.

14. Andrews P, Sinclair L, Harris B, et al. Study of therapeutic hypothermia for intracranial pressure reduction after traumatic brain injury: outcome of the pilot phase of the trial. Trials 2013;14:277.

15. Sadaka F, Veremakis C. Therapeutic hypothermia for the management of intracranial hypertension in severe traumatic brain injury: a systematic review. Brain Inj 2012;26(7–8):899–908.

16. Patel K, Kokias A, Hutchinson P. What's new in the surgical management of traumatic brain injury. J Neurol 2015;262:235–8.

17. Grandhi R, Bonfield C, Newman W, et al. Surgical management of traumatic brain injury: a review of guidelines, pathophysiology, neurophysiology, outcomes, and controversies. J Neurosurg Sci 2014;58(4):249–59.

18. Bor-Seng-Shu E, Figueiredo E, Foneff E, et al. Decompressive craniectomy and head injury: brain morphometry, ICP, cerebral hemodynamics, cerebral microvascular reactivity, and neurochemistry. Neurosurg Rev 2013;36(3):361–70.

19. Bor-Seng-Shu E, Figueiredo E, Amorim R, et al. Decompressive craniectomy: a meta-analysis of influences on intracranial pressure and cerebral perfusion pressure in the treatment of traumatic brain injury. J Neurosurg 2012;117:589–96.

20. Cooper D, Rosenfeld J, Murray L, et al. Decompressive craniectomy in diffuse traumatic brain injury. N Engl J Med 2011;364(16):1493–502.

21. Nirula R, Millar D, Greene T, et al. Decompressive craniectomy or medical management for refractory intracranial hypertension: an AAST-MIT propensity score analysis. J Trauma Acute Care Surg 2014;76(4):944–52.

22. Chibbaro S, Di Rocco F, Mirone G, et al. Decompressive craniectomy and early cranioplasty for the management of severe head injury: a prospective multicenter study on 147 patients. World Neurosurg 2011;75(3–4):558–62.

23. Honeybul S, Ho K. Decompressive craniectomy for severe traumatic brain injury: the relationship between surgical complications and the prediction of an unfavorable outcome. Injury 2014;45:1332–9.

24. Ahmadi S, Meier U, Lemcke J. Detailed long-term outcome analysis after decompressive craniectomy for severe traumatic brain injury. Brain Inj 2010;24(13–14): 1539–49.

25. Honeybul S, Janzen C, Kruger K, et al. Decompressive craniectomy for severe traumatic brain injury: is life worth living? J Neurosurg 2013;119:1566–75.

26. Basheer N, Gupta D, Mahapatra A, et al. Cranioplasty following decompressive craniectomy in traumatic brain injury: experience at level I apex trauma centre. The Indian Journal of Neurotrauma 2010;7(2):139–44.

27. Tasiou A, Vagkopoulos K, Georgiadis I, et al. Cranioplasty optimal timing in cases of decompressive craniectomy after severe head injury: a systematic literature review. Interdisciplinary Neurosurgery 2014;1(4):107–11.

28. Chien P, Khan K, Arnott N. Magnesium sulphate in the treatment of eclampsia and pre-eclampsia: an overview of the evidence from randomised trials. Br J Obstet Gynaecol 1996;103(11):1085–91.
29. Lu J, Nightingale C. Magnesium sulfate in eclampsia and pre-eclampsia: pharmacokinetic principles. Clin Pharmacokinet 2000;38(4):305–14.
30. Temkin N, Anderson G, Winn H, et al. Magnesium sulfate for neuroprotection after traumatic brain injury: a randomised controlled trial. Lancet Neurol 2007;6(1): 29–38.
31. The CRASH trial management group. The CRASH trial protocol (Corticosteroid Randomization after Significant Head Injury). BMC Emerg Med 2001;1(1):1. Available at: http://www.biomedcentral.com/141-227x1/1.
32. Alderson P, Roberts I. Corticosteroids for acute traumatic brain injury. Cochrane Database Syst Rev 2009;(1):CD000196.
33. Wright D, Kellermann A, Hertzberg V, et al. ProTECT: a randomized clinical trial of progesterone for acute traumatic brain injury. Ann Emerg Med 2003;20(10):1–13.
34. Xiao G, Wei J, Yan W, et al. Improved outcomes from the administration of progesterone for patients with acute sever traumatic brain injury: a randomized controlled trial. Crit Care 2008;12:R61.
35. Leibowitz A, Boyko M, Shapira Y, et al. Blood glutamate scavenging: insight into neuroprotection. Int J Mol Sci 2012;13:10041–66.
36. Zlotnik A, Sinnelnikov I, Gruenbaum B, et al. Effect of glutamate and blood glutamate scavengers oxaloacetate and pyruvate on neurological outcome and pathohistology of the hippocampus after traumatic injury in rats. Anesthesiology 2012; 116(1):73–83.
37. Liu SP, Fu RH, Huang SJ, et al. Stem cell applications in regenerative medicine for neurological disorders. Cell Transplant 2013;22:631–7.
38. Mouhieddine T, Kobeissy F, Itani M, et al. Stem cells in neuroinjury and neurodegenerative disorders: challenges and future neurotherapeutic prospects. Neural Regen Res 2014;9(9):901–6.

Pain Management in Military Trauma

Kim Litwack, PhD, RN, FAAN, APNP[a,b,*]

KEYWORDS

- Military trauma • Military pain management • Battlefield pain management
- War injury pain management • War zone pain management

KEY POINTS

- Battlefield pain management is difficult given both the situation and the personnel involved.
- The management of acute pain may help prevent the development of chronic pain and post-traumatic stress disorder.
- Pain management strategies range from self-care in the field to implantable therapies following medical discharge.

INTRODUCTION

Although military health care has been criticized of late related to tardiness and lack of timely access to health care, battlefield medicine has been exemplary in care, with a 90% survival rate.[1] The nation expects no less than outstanding care of for its warriors, and the respect given to servicemen and women is at a new high. A report from the Office of the Army Surgeon General on pain management and care for military members and their families states:

> "While trauma management has been at the forefront of excellence, pain management associated with combat polytrauma provides unique challenges because of the distinctive mission, structure, and patient population of the military casualty patient. The transient nature of the military population, including patients and providers, makes continuity of care a challenge to military medicine."[2(pE2)]

Much of what is known about pain management in the trauma patient in the nonmilitary population, both pharmacologic and nonpharmacologic has not found its way

Disclosure Statement: Nothing to disclose.
[a] University of Wisconsin-Milwaukee College of Nursing, 1921 East Hartford Avenue, Milwaukee, WI 53201, USA; [b] Advanced Pain Management, 34 Schroeder Ct, Madison, WI 53711, USA
* Corresponding author.
E-mail address: litwack@uwm.edu

into military trauma management, where the priority has always been on improving survivability.[2]

In 2009, the Army Surgeon General, Lt. Gen. Eric B. Schoomaker, chartered an Army Pain Management Task Force to make recommendations for a US Army Medical Command (MEDCOM) comprehensive pain management strategy that was holistic, multidisciplinary, and multimodal in its approach; that utilized state of the art/science modalities and technologies; and that provided optimal quality of life for soldiers and other patients with acute and chronic pain.[2(pE1,2)]

The Pain Management Task Force came back with 109 recommendations, in 4 areas, that led to a comprehensive pain management strategy that met the directives (**Box 1**).

In 2010, the National Defense Authorization Act continued the initiative by tasking the secretary of defense with developing and implementing a comprehensive policy on pain management by the Military Health Service no later than March 31, 2011.[2(pE2)]

The policy had 7 specific targets, noted in **Box 2**.

It should be noted that a focus on pain assessment and management was not new to the US military. In 1998, the Veterans Health Administration (VHA) initiated a national pain strategy in an effort to develop a system-wide approach to pain management, with the ultimate goal of reducing suffering among veterans with acute and chronic pain. "Pain as the 5th vital sign" was promoted in all inpatient and outpatient clinical settings in order to ensure consistency of pain assessments throughout the VHA. This initiative migrated into civilian health care settings.[2]

This initiative was strengthened in 2009, with a VHA directive for pain management.

This directive provided policy and implementation procedures for the improvement of pain management consistent with the VHA National Pain Management Strategy and in compliance with generally accepted pain management standards of care. It also defined the stepped care model for pain management. Stepped care balances a focus on managing pain as early as possible in a primary care setting while providing access to pain medicine specialty consultation, and interdisciplinary and multimodal pain management resources when required. It also emphasizes optimal pain control, improved function, and improved quality of life.[2(p9)]

In 2000, the Joint Commission on Accreditation for Healthcare Organizations (JCAHO) unveiled pain management standards that become an accreditation assessment criteria for all JCAHO-accredited ambulatory care facilities, behavioral health

---

Box 1
Pain Management task force target areas

1. Provide tools and infrastructure that support and encourage practice and research advancements in pain management

2. Build a full spectrum of best practices for the continuum of acute and chronic pain, based on a foundation of best available evidence

3. Focus on the warrior and family, sustaining the force

4. Synchronize a culture of pain awareness, education and proactive intervention

From United States. Office of the Army Surgeon General. Pain management task force: final report—providing a standardized DoD and VHA vision and approach to pain management to optimize the care for warriors and their families. Washington, DC: 2010. E1–2.

Box 2
National Defense Authorization Act comprehensive pain management policy

1. Management of acute and chronic pain

2. Standard of care for pain management to be used throughout the Department of Defense

3. The consistent application of pain assessments throughout the Department of Defense

4. The assurance of prompt and appropriate pain care treatment and management by the department when medically necessary

5. Programs of research related to acute and chronic pain, including pain attributable to central and peripheral nervous system damage characteristic of injuries incurred in modern warfare, brain injuries, and chronic migraine headache

6. Programs of pain care education and training for health care personnel of the Department of Defense

7. An assessment of the dissemination of information on pain management to beneficiaries enrolled in the military health care system.

From United States. Office of the Army Surgeon General. Pain management task force: final report—providing a standardized DoD and VHA vision and approach to pain management to optimize the care for warriors and their families. Washington, DC: 2010. E2.

---

care organizations, critical access hospitals, home care providers, hospitals, office-based surgery practices, and long-term care providers. The pain management standards address the assessment and management of pain, requiring organizations to

- Recognize the right of patients to appropriate assessment and management of pain
- Screen patients for pain during their initial assessment, and, when clinically required, during ongoing, periodic reassessments
- Educate patients suffering from pain and their families about pain management[3]

One consistent theme in all of these initiatives was the recognition of suffering, and the attention to the continuum of pain management as a means to promote recovery, rehabilitation as needed and overall quality of life. In the case of the military, it may include return to duty or transition to discharge. Pain, if poorly managed, adversely affects every aspect of a soldier's recovery and rehabilitation.[2] Consequences of un-relieved pain are well documented and researched, to include both physiologic responses in almost every organ system, as well as psychological consequences. As stated in an article by Bowman and colleagues

> *"Early pain control has become an increasingly crucial prehospital military task and must be controlled from the pain-initiating event. Inadequate early pain control may lead to a range of changes in blood pressure to delayed wound healing and posttraumatic stress disorder."*[4(pS43)]

The continuum of pain management for the soldier begins with wounding, and continues through the chain of evacuation to rehabilitation, with the result being either continued employment in the service or medical discharge.[5] Aldington referred to this continuum as "end to end military pain management".[6]

BATTLEFIELD PAIN MANAGEMENT

Pain management in combat situations exacerbates the typical challenges found in treating acute pain and has the additional obstacles of a lack of supplies and equipment, delayed or prolonged evacuation times and distances, devastating injuries, provider inexperience, and dangerous tactical situations. These factors contribute to the difficulty of controlling a soldier's pain in combat.[7(p223)]

Research has confirmed that battlefield pain care has been less than optimal because of a lack of equipment and inadequate provider training in pain management, resulting in an over-reliance on opioid-based pain solutions, from the point of injury throughout the care continuum.[8]

It will be the continued purpose of this article to discuss both the current, as well as emerging pain management strategies for the battlefield trauma patient.

MINOR PAIN: MELOXICAM AND ACETAMINOPHEN

Battlefield pain of a minor nature is self-managed with the use of meloxicam and acetaminophen (Table 1). Now part of the Tactical Combat Casualty Care (TCCC) guidelines, the use of these medications was initially challenged with concern that soldiers would manage pain without reporting injury. As soldiers were found to effectively manage minor pains with these medications, without untoward effects, the medications are now considered first-line therapy for minor pain, including headache or musculoskeletal discomforts. These 2 medications are the most common medications carried by service members in combat situations.[7]

The combat medic has access to additional analgesics, both opioid and nonopioid, for use if the service member can no longer remain in combat.[9]

OPIOID THERAPY—MORPHINE

Morphine administration has served as the primary method of battlefield pain management since the American Civil War.[8] Although effective and easily administered via intramuscular injection, this therapy is associated with unpredictable results and adverse effects. Intramuscular administration is selected as it is fast, but the vasoconstriction that is often associated with significant trauma makes its absorption unpredictable in terms of onset. Starting an intravenous line when the goal is immediate evacuation results in a delay of care, yet intravenous or interosseous access, will be the mainstay for fluid resuscitation.

Morphine also causes adverse effects of respiratory depression, sedation, nausea, and vomiting, which may prove fatal to persons wounded in combat.[8] In addition, the need for personnel to manage these complications puts additional personnel at risk.

OPIOID THERAPY—ORAL TRANSMUCOSAL FENTANYL CITRATE

In 2014, Aldington reported on the introduction of transmucosal fentanyl citrate as a battlefield option. The 400 μg dose was selected for study, as this dose has been

Table 1 Meloxicam and acetaminophen actions		
Drug	**Mechanism of Action**	**Effects**
Meloxicam	Prostaglandin (cycloxygenase) inhibition	Anti-inflammatory Analgesic
	Inhibition of prostaglandins	Antipyretic
Acetaminophen	Inhibition of nitric oxide pathway including N-methyl-D-aspartate (NMDA) and substance P	Analgesic
	Inhibition of pyrogens, blocking of prostaglandins	Antipyretic

used clinically in the opiate-naive patient. The 400 μg dose is clinically equivalent to the 4 to 8 mg intravenous dose and 10 mg intramuscular morphine dose used as standard practice. Its advantages in a combat situation include its ease of administration, as well as its usefulness in parenteral administration, deemed essential to allow for use in chemical, biological, radiological, and nuclear contaminated environments.[6,8]

Although the fentanyl lozenge met the desired criteria, initial clinical use has been limited by a lack of understanding of clinicians in the pharmacokinetics and pharmacodynamics of the drug and delivery system, the significant adverse effects of nausea and vomiting, and variable efficacy. One significant finding was the absence of respiratory depression at the trial dose.[10]

Wedmore (2012)[11] reported on the use of oral transmucosal fentanyl citrate (OTFC) for prehospital pain control in a battlefield setting, finding a significant reduction in pain intensity at time of administration, sustained at 15 and 30 minutes after the traumatic event. Only 18.2% of patients required other types of analgesics. Nausea was the most significant adverse effect. OTFC was seen as a safe and effective alternative for the prehospital battlefield setting, particularly because of its usefulness in austere environments.[11]

Implemented in 2012, Tactical Combat Casualty Care (TCCC) guidelines now call for the use of OTFC for casualties who are unable to continue fighting when interosseous or intravenous access cannot be established. Morphine intramuscularly remains the standard for use when interosseous and/or intravenous access can be easily obtained.[12]

ANESTHETIC AS ANALGESIC THERAPY: KETAMINE

The administration of intranasal and intramuscular ketamine is another agent considered for battlefield use. Ketamine is classified as a dissociative anesthetic, but one with hallucinogenic and psychoactive properties. It has been used as the sole anesthetic for short painful procedures, such as orthopedic splinting, laceration repair, or fracture resetting. Ketamine offers the advantages of profound pain relief, while maintaining airway reflexes and stimulating cardiac function. It acts as a mild sedative and produces a sense of euphoria.[13] Current Tactical Combat Casualty Care (TCCC) guidelines have incorporated the use of intramuscular ketamine for battlefield trauma, except in patients with traumatic brain injury or open globe injuries. This is out of concern that ketamine has been associated with increased intracranial pressure and increased intraocular pressure. Current research, however, challenges thinking about ketamine's effect on intracranial pressure and intraocular pressure.[14,15] This is not based on clinical trial or study in a battlefield setting, but initiated after significant interdisciplinary study by the Defense Health Board to the Department of Defense, in recognition that ketamine offers the benefits of significant pain control without opioid-induced hypotension or respiratory depression.[16]

During Operation Enduring Freedom in Afghanistan, the 82nd Airborne Division, followed by the 3rd Infantry Division and then the 4th Infantry Division, piloted the use of intranasal ketamine on the battlefield with wounded service members. Intranasal ketamine use has been established in peer-reviewed clinical practice guidelines based in primary literature.[16]

ADDITIONAL PAIN THERAPIES: ACUPUNCTURE, REGIONAL BLOCKS, EPIDURALS

Commonplace in civilian pain management, the use of acupuncture and trigger point injections, regional nerve blocks, and epidural analgesia has now found its way into military pain management. Although not extensively used, Hommer reported on the use of scalp acupuncture to relieve pain and to restore function in complex regional pain syndromes.[17] This is a particularly important finding, as nerve injuries are a significant trauma finding in battlefield injuries, with prolonged conduction block/neuropraxia, axonotmesis, and neurotmesis being outcomes of explosive injury.[18]

Interventional analgesia, as part of an acute pain management service trialed in Afghanistan, used trigger point injections, as well as the use of regional nerve blocks and epidural analgesia, as a means to decrease pain intensity, to provide increased pain relief, and to avoid the adverse effects associated with opioid therapy.[19] This may prove particularly beneficial in the management of postamputation pain, where phantom limb sensations were more effectively treated with early regional blockade.[20]

Continuous peripheral nerve blocks, including placement of continuous transversus abdominis plane catheters, demonstrated that advanced regional anesthesia could be accomplished in a forward deployed environment. Although current evidence concerning battlefield use is limited, common combat wounds, namely traumatic amputations, are compatible with this technique.[21–23]

Use of these advanced techniques requires the integration of appropriately trained personnel as part of the front line team.[24] Pain management, as part of trauma management, must be firmly embedded in warfare casualty management with responsible practitioners firmly established in using the process.[24,25]

CONTINUED PAIN MANAGEMENT FOLLOWING STABILIZATION

Although pain management on the battlefield is the immediate priority, once stabilized, casualties not able to return to the battlefield will be evacuated for long-term management and rehabilitation. As 90% of wounded soldiers survive their injuries, continued care and management have become priorities. The transition to outpatient care will require stabilizing the patient on pain medications that are appropriate for an outpatient setting. Although opioid therapy (at times high dose and/or parenteral) is appropriate for acute pain, transition to outpatient and ambulatory care for continued and chronic pain will become a priority. The comprehensive interventional pain clinic has become a vital component of the medical treatment system built for the comprehensive care of every service member.[26]

Ongoing pain management will use a holistic approach, integrating care of the body and mind in pain management. This will include pharmacologic and nonpharmacologic therapies.

PHARMACOLOGIC THERAPIES: OPIOIDS
Short- and Long-Acting Oral Agents

Opioids are indicated for the management of moderate-to-severe pain. Short-acting opioids, for moderate-to-severe pain of an intermittent nature, may respond well to opioids with a limited duration of action, such as hydrocodone or oxycodone. Both agents are limited to a 4- to 6 -hour duration of action. Oral transmucosal fentanyl citrate is an ultrashort-acting medication for severe breakthrough pain, and it is most commonly used in terminal illness.

Long-acting opioids, with an 8- to 12-hour duration of action, can be used to stabilize the patient requiring around-the-clock pain management, to avoid the peaks and valleys associated with the use of short-acting medications. Long-acting medications include morphine, methadone, oxymorphone, oxycontin, hydromorphone, and tapentadol. Methadone and tapentadol offer the advantage of also having success in the control of neuropathic pain.[27,28] Methadone requires particular care in use, as it is associated with prolongation of the QT interval and torsade de pointes.[29,30]

Methadone use requires a baseline electrocardiogram (EKG) and yearly EKG monitoring. Of benefit, military personnel, at least on initial medical discharge, are likely to be younger and healthy, and better able to tolerate any conduction changes. All of these agents have the advantage of being able to be delivered orally, making them useful in the outpatient setting.

Transdermal Agents

Fentanyl and buprenorphine, two other long-acting medications, are delivered most commonly by a transdermal delivery system (patch). Fentanyl patches are traditionally changed every 72 hours; buprenorphine patches are changed every 7 days.

Intrathecal

Although oral and transdermal use is the most common, intrathecal delivery systems (pain pumps) can be used for intractable pain that is unresponsive to more traditional therapies. Opioids can be used as sole agents, or in combination with local anesthetics such as bupivicaine, with muscle relaxants such as baclofen, and with other adjuvants, such as clonidine. Only the use of morphine, baclofen, and ziconitide are approved by the US Food and Drug Administration for use. The others, alone or in combination therapy, are off-label use.[31]

Intrathecal opioids work by binding to opiate receptors in the substantia gelatinosa of the dorsal horn of the spinal cord, a major site for the integration of nociceptive input.[32]

PHARMACOLOGIC THERAPIES: NEUROMODULATORS
Gabapentin, Duloxetine, and Pregabalin

Although opioids are the mainstay of acute pain management, adjuvant therapies, including gabapentin, cymbalta, and pregabalin, have found a place in the management of chronic neuropathic pain associated with nerve trauma. Not started on the battlefield, studies confirm early use to stabilize damaged nerves can help to prevent the chronicity of long-term incapacitating neuropathic pain.

Gabapentin, originally used as an anticonvulsant, has proven useful in nerve damage and nerve trauma and phantom limb pain, although its exact mode of action is not well understood. Theories include reduction of membrane excitability, enhancing synapse inhibition, and decreasing nerve conduction across calcium channels.[33]

Duloxetine is a centrally acting analgesic with selective 5-HT and norepinephrine reuptake inhibition. Studies have confirmed its usefulness in not only neuropathic conditions, but in central pain syndromes, chronic low back pain, and inflammatory disorders.[34–36]

Pregabalin relieves pain caused by damage to nerves, either from injury or disease by rebalancing neurotransmitters involved in central pain amplification. This medication has proven useful in chronic neuropathic pain, but there is no evidence to support its use in acute pain management.[37]

PHARMACOLOGIC THERAPIES: ANTIDEPRESSANTS
Pain and Post-traumatic Stress Disorder

It has long been recognized that healing of the body is embedded in the healing of the mind, spirit, and soul. Increased pain is associated with increased anxiety, distress, and worry, suggesting the need for psychological management along with analgesia.[38] The US Army Institute of Surgical Research asserts:

"Predisposing factors for PTSD include experiencing a traumatic event, threat of injury or death, and untreated pain; thus almost all deployed service members are

at risk for PTSD. Randomized clinical trials of patients whose pain is either adequately controlled or inadequately controlled are not ethical or practical to determine the effect of analgesics and pain control on PTSD development."[39]

The active use of spiritual care providers and pain management psychologists to minimize disability and post-traumatic stress has received increasing attention. An article on depression and pain in Harvard Health Publications states:

"Pain, especially chronic pain, is a complex experience that affects thought, mood, and behavior and can lead to isolation, anxiety, and depression. Patients with chronic pain have three times the average risk of developing psychiatric symptoms of mood and anxiety disorders, and depressed patients have three times the average risk of developing chronic pain."[40]

Medications may be used to treat depression and anxiety, particularly when there is concern about a service member self-medicating with alcohol and other prescribed or illegal substances. Relieving anxiety, fatigue, depression or insomnia associated with chronic pain will also ease chronic pain.[41] **Table 2** lists the types of common antidepressants used in the management of pain.

Tricyclic Antidepressants

Major classes of antidepressants used to treat depression have different roles in the treatment of pain. Tricyclic antidepressants such as amitriptyline and nortriptyline heighten the activity of the neurotransmitters norepinephrine and serotonin. Their sedative properties are also useful in managing the insomnia that frequently accompanies pain, improving sleep and rest.[42] Although effective, these medications are associated with a greater risk of misuse and have a lower margin of safety.[43,44]

SELECTIVE SEROTONIN REUPTAKE INHIBITORS

Selective serotonin reuptake inhibitors (SSRIs) manage depression and its associated anxiety, thereby helping to reduce the distress of pain. These agents act selectively on serotonin.

SELECTIVE NORADRENALINE (NOREPINEPHRINE) REUPTAKE INHIBITORS

Serotonin noradrenaline reuptake inhibitors (SNRIs) are also called dual-action agents, as they block the reuptake of both serotonin and noradrenaline. SNRIs have a third action, increasing dopamine in the prefrontal cortex, thereby treating both depression and anxiety. The mechanisms underlying this role of action include inhibition of serotonin and norepinephrine reuptake, leading to enhanced descending inhibition of centrally sensitized pain.[45,46]

Table 2
Common antidepressants used in pain management

Tricyclic Antidepressants	SSRI	SNRI
Amitriptyline	Citalopram	Duloxetine
Nortriptyline	Escitalopram	Venlafaxine
Imipramine	Fluoxetine	Desvenlafaxine
Desipramine	Paroxetine	
	Sertraline	

NONPHARMACOLOGIC THERAPIES
Interventional Techniques: Nerve Blocks and Rhizotomy

There are times, and types of pain, for which the use of medication therapy is not tolerated because of adverse effects, or is ineffective because of the type of pain. Interventional pain management, to include the use of nerve blocks, provides powerful, albeit temporary, pain relief through the injection of steroid and/or local anesthetics to the site of pain. A semipermanent intervention, through the use of radiofrequency nerve ablation, also known as radiofrequency rhizotomy, has been employed in the management of facet-mediated back pain, spinal stenosis, and trigeminal neuralgia.[47,48]

Interventional Techniques: Neuromodulation

Therapeutic neuromodulation is defined as the alteration of nerve activity through the delivery of electrical stimulation or chemical agents to targeted sites of the body.[49] In use since the 1980s, neuromodulation stimulates nerves in such as way as to alter abnormal nerve pathways caused by a disease process or injury. A fully reversible therapy, neuromodulation delivers stimulation to specific neural circuits in the brain, spine, or peripheral nerves. Neuromodulation ranges from external, noninvasive techniques such as transcutaneous electrical nerve stimulator (TENS) therapy and transcranial magnetic stimulation, to more invasive, implanted therapies such as spinal cord stimulation for neuropathic pain, including complex regional pain syndrome, which may develop after a traumatic injury.[50,51]

Physical and Occupational Therapy

Physical therapy as part of rehabilitation is designed to assist individuals with the achievement, maintenance, and restoration of maximal physical functioning, with the secondary goal of minimizing disability.[52] The goal of occupational therapy is help individuals to increase their functional independence in daily life while preventing or minimizing disability.[53]

Complementary and Alternative Therapies

The Pain Management Task Force of the Army Office of the Surgeon General called for an increased use of complementary and alternative medicine (CAM) as an adjuvant therapy to pharmaceutical agents. Acupuncture was trialed on the battlefield. It is thought that acupuncture helps to control pain by stimulating specific acupuncture points with nonpainful impulses transmitted to the spinal cord to block C fiber transmission for pain relief.[52]

Another therapy under investigation is the use of immersion virtual reality (VR) during painful procedures to reduce pain nonpharmacologically. Researchers consistently reported 30% to 50% reductions in pain ratings when VR was used during severe burn wound care.[53]

Yoga has been included in the management of osteoarthritis and low back pain to reduce pain and disability, while improving strength, balance, and gait.[54]

Massage therapy has had conflicting results as an adjunctive pain management strategy. It appears to have a more lasting benefit on psychological distress more so than the physical perception of pain.

The research on herbal therapy for pain management is limited, as there is little incentive on the part of pharmaceutical companies to engage clinical trials; additionally, doing so is costly for companies producing herbal therapies that are not subject to FDA regulation. A review of the literature does identify the use of fish oil, tumeric, green tea, ginger, rosemary, cat's claw, devil's claw, and willow bark as having pain control and in some cases (willow bark) antipyretic properties.[55–57]

SUMMARY

Although battlefield survivability has steadily improved, it was not until 2009 that pain management of the wounded warrior became a directed military initiative, recognizing that early pain management is critical to a service member's recovery and rehabilitation. Beginning with wounding, carrying forward to either a return to duty, or to medical discharge, care of the wounded service member is directed toward relieving physical as well as psychological distress. This requires the use of multimodal therapies, and a comprehensive pain management program.

REFERENCES

1. Buckenmaier CC 3rd, Brandon-Edwards H, Borden D Jr, et al. Treating pain on the battlefield: a warrior's perspective. Curr Pain Headache Rep 2010;14(1):1–7.
2. Office of the Army Surgeon General. Pain management task force: final report—providing a standardized DoD and VHA vision and approach to pain management to optimize the care for warriors and their families. Washington, DC: 2010. p. E1–2, 9, 26.
3. Available at: http://www.jointcommission.org/pain_management/. Accessed November 13, 2014.
4. Bowman WJ, Nesbitt ME, Therien SP. The effects of standardized trauma training on prehospital pain control: have pain medication administration rates increased on the battlefield? J Trauma Acute Care Surg 2012;73(2 Suppl 1):S43–8.
5. Aldington D. Pain management in victims of conflict. Curr Opin Support Palliat Care 2012;6(2):172–6.
6. Aldington DJ, McQuay HJ, Moore RA. End-to-end military pain management. Philos Trans R Soc Lond B Biol Sci 2011;366(1562):268–75.
7. Black IH, McManus J. Pain management in current combat operations [abstract]. Prehosp Emerg Care 2009;13(2):223–7.
8. Buckenmaier CC 3rd. The role of pain management in recovery following trauma and orthopaedic surgery. J Am Acad Orthop Surg 2012;20(Suppl 1):S35–8.
9. Malchow RJ, Black IH. The evolution of pain management in the critically ill trauma patient: emerging concepts from the global war on terrorism. Crit Care Med 2008;36(7 Suppl):S346–57.
10. Aldington D, Jagdish S. The fentanyl 'lozenge' story: from books to battlefield. J R Army Med Corps 2014;160(2):102–4.
11. Wedmore IS, Kotwal RS, McManus JG, et al. Safety and efficacy of oral transmucosal fentanyl citrate for prehospital pain control on the battlefield. J Trauma Acute Care Surg 2012;73(6 Suppl 5):S490–5.
12. Available at: http://www.itstactical.com/medcom/tccc-medcom/2014-tccc-tactical-combat-casualty-care-guidelines/. Accessed November 13, 2014.
13. Green SM, Roback MG, Kennedy RM, et al. Clinical practice guideline for emergency department ketamine dissociative sedation: 2011 update. Ann Emerg Med 2011;57:449–63.
14. Filanovsky Y, Miller P, Kao J, et al. Myth: ketamine should not be used as an induction agent for intubation in patients with head injury. CJEM 2010;12(2):152–7.
15. Drayna PC, Estrada C, Wang W, et al. Ketamine is not associated with elevation of intraocular pressure during procedural sedation. Am J Emerg Med 2012;30(7):1215–8.

16. Defense Health Board report to the DoD: prehospital use of ketamine in battlefield analgesia 2012-03. Available at: http://www.health.mil/~/media/MHS/Report%20Files/201203.ashx. Accessed November 13, 2014.
17. Hommer DH. Chinese scalp acupuncture relieves pain and restores function in complex regional pain syndrome. Mil Med 2012;177(10):1231–4.
18. Birch R, Misra P, Stewart MP, et al. Nerve injuries sustained during warfare: Part I-Epidemiology. J Bone Joint Surg Br 2012;94(4):523–8.
19. Buckenmaier C 3rd, Mahoney PF, Anton T, et al. Impact of an acute pain service on pain outcomes with combat-inured soldiers at Camp Bastion Afghanistan. Pain Med 2012;13(7):919–26.
20. Aldington D, Small C, Edwards D, et al. A survey of post-amputation pains in serving military personnel. J R Army Med Corps 2014;160(1):38–41.
21. Hunter JG. Managing pain on the battlefield: an introduction to continuous peripheral nerve blocks. J R Army Med Corps 2010;156(4):230–2.
22. Allcock E, Spencer E, Frazer R, et al. Continuous transversus abdominis plane (TAP) block catheters in a combat surgical environment. Pain Med 2010;11(9):1426–9.
23. Caruso JD, Elster EA, Rodriguez CJ, et al. Epidural placement does not result in an increased incidence of venous thromboembolism in combat-wounded patients. J Trauma Acute Care Surg 2014;77(1):61–6.
24. Buckenmaier CC. Interview: 21st century battlefield pain management. Pain Manag 2013;3(4):269–75.
25. Birch R, Misra P, Stewart MP, et al. Nerve injuries sustained during warfare: Part II: outcomes. J Bone Joint Surg Br 2012;94(4):529–35.
26. Clifford JL, Fowler M, Hansen JJ, et al. State of the science review: advances in pain management in wounded service members over a decade at war. J Trauma Acute Care Surg 2014;77(3 Suppl 2):S228–36.
27. Morley JS, Bridson J, Nash TP, et al. Low-dose methadone has an analgesic effect in neuropathic pain: a double-blind randomized controlled crossover trial. Palliat Med 2003;17(7):576–87.
28. Kress HG. Tapentadol and its two mechanisms of action: is there a new pharmacological class of centrally-acting analgesics on the horizon? Eur J Pain 2010;14(8):781–3.
29. Keane H. Categorising methadone: addiction and analgesia. Int J Drug Policy 2013;24:e18–24.
30. Stringer J. Methadone-associated Q-T interval prolongation and torsade de pointes. Am J Health Syst Pharm 2009;66(9):825–33.
31. Bennett G, Serafini M, Burchiel K, et al. Evidence-based review of the literature on intrathecal drug delivery of pain medication. J Pain Symptom Manage 2000; 20(2):S12–36.
32. Herkenham M, Pert CB. Light microscopic localization of brain opiate receptors: a general auto-radiographic method which preserves tissue quality. J Neurosci 1982;2:1120–49.
33. Moore RA, Wiffen PJ, Derry S, et al. Gabapentin for chronic neuropathic pain and fibromyalgia in adults. Cochrane Database Syst Rev 2014;(4):CD007938.
34. Mease PJ, Walker DJ, Alaka K. Evaluation of duloxetine for chronic pain conditions. Pain Manag 2011;1(2):159–70.
35. Skljarevski V, Ossanna M, Liu-Seifert H, et al. A double-blind, randomized trial of duloxetine versus placebo in the management of chronic low back pain. Eur J Neurol 2009;16(9):1041–8.
36. Chappell AS, Desaiah D, Liu-Seifert H, et al. A double-blind, randomized, placebo-controlled study of the efficacy and safety of duloxetine for the treatment of chronic pain due to osteoarthritis of the knee. Pain Pract 2011;11(1):33–41.

37. Moore RA, Straube S, Wiffen PJ, et al. Pregabalin for acute and chronic pain in adults (Review). Cochrane Database Syst Rev 2010;2009(3):CD007076.
38. Buckenmaier CC 3rd, Rupprecht C, McKnight G, et al. Pain following battlefield injury and evacuation: a survey of 110 casualties from the wars in Iraq and Afghanistan. Pain Med 2009;10(8):1487–96.
39. US Army Institute of Surgical Research. Battlefield pain management. Available at: http://www.usaisr.amedd.army.mil/battle_pain_management.html. Accessed November 13, 2014.
40. Available at: http://www.health.harvard.edu/newsweek/Depression_and_pain.htm. Accessed November 20, 2014.
41. Lynch EM. Antidepressants as analgesics: a review of randomised controlled trials. J Psychiatry Neurosci 2001;26:30–6.
42. Ferjan I, Lipnik-Stangelj M. Chronic pain treatment: the influence of tricyclic antidepressants on serotonin release and uptake in mast cells. Mediators Inflamm 2013;2013:340473.
43. Frommer DA, Kulig KW, Marx JA, et al. Tricyclic antidepressant overdose. A review. JAMA 1987;257(4):521–6.
44. Kerr GW, McGuffie AC, Wilkie S. Tricyclic antidepressant overdose: a review. Emerg Med J 2001;18(4):236–41.
45. Stahl SM, Grady MM, Moret C, et al. SNRIs: their pharmacology, clinical efficacy, and tolerability in comparison with other classes of antidepressants. CNS Spectr 2005;10(9):732–47.
46. Marks DM, Shah MJ, Patkar AA, et al. Serotonin-Norepinephrine reuptake inhibitors for pain control: premise and promise. Curr Neuropharmacol 2009;7(4):331–6.
47. Bogduk N, Dreyfuss P, Govind J. A narrative review of lumbar medial branch neurotomy for the treatment of back pain. Pain Med 2009;10(6):1035–45.
48. Taha JM, Tew JM. Comparison of surgical treatments for trigeminal neuralgia: reevaluation of radiofrequency rhizotomy. Neurosurgery 1996;38(5):865–71.
49. International Neuromodulation Society. Welcome to the International Neuromodulation Society. Available at: www.neuromodulation.com. Accessed November 20, 2014.
50. Taylor RS, Van Buyten JP, Buchser E. Spinal cord stimulation for complex regional pain syndrome: a systematic review of the clinical and cost effectiveness literature and assessment of prognostic factors. Eur J Pain 2006;10(2):91–101.
51. Mekhail NA, Cheng J, Narouze S, et al. Clinical applications of neurostimulation: forty years later. Pain Pract 2010;10(2):103–12.
52. American Physical Therapy Association. Guide to physical therapist practice. 2nd edition. Alexandria (Egypt): American Physical Therapy Association; 2003.
53. American Occupational Therapy Association. Standards of practice for occupational therapy. Am J Occup Ther 2005;59:663–5.
54. Man PL, Chen CH. Mechanism of acupunctural anesthesia: the two-gate control theory. Dis Nerv Syst 1972;33(11):730–5.
55. Hoffman HG, Patterson DR, Seibel E, et al. Virtual reality pain control during burn wound debridement in the hydrotank. Clin J Pain 2008;24(4):299–304.
56. Ebnezar J, Nagarathna R, Yogitha B, et al. Effects of an integrated approach of hatha yoga therapy on functional disability, pain and flexibility in osteoarthritis of the knee joint: a randomized controlled study. J Altern Complement Med 2012;18(5):463–72.
57. US Department of Health and Human Services, National Institute of Health, National Center for Complementary and Alternative Medicine (NCCAM). Available at: http://nccam.nih.gov/. Accessed November 20, 2014.

Evidence-based Treatments for Military-related Posttraumatic Stress Disorder in a Veterans Affairs Setting

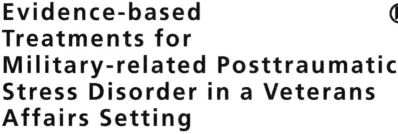

Scott A. Driesenga, PhD*, Jessica L. Rodriguez, PhD,
Thomas Picard, MD

KEYWORDS

- Veterans • Posttraumatic stress disorder • PTSD • Evidence-based treatment
- Outcomes

KEY POINTS

- Posttraumatic stress disorder has a significant negative impact on the physical, emotional, and mental health of individuals.
- Posttraumatic stress disorder has a high prevalence in the Veteran population.
- Thorough assessment of posttraumatic stress disorder is essential, and evidence-based treatments for posttraumatic stress disorder are very effective.
- A collaborative approach between primary care and mental health providers is critical.
- Many posttraumatic stress disorder symptoms respond quite well to appropriate psycho-pharmacologic intervention.

INTRODUCTION

Posttraumatic stress disorder (PTSD) is a debilitating disorder that impacts upwards of 30% of Veterans in their lifetimes. Fortunately, there are several effective treatments identified that have been shown to decrease symptoms and improve quality of life. Given that many Veterans with PTSD first present to primary care settings, it is important to consider the role of PCPs in the initial assessment of symptoms, delivery of care, and referral process. The purpose of this article is to describe the salient features of PTSD, the assessment and treatment of PTSD with a special focus on the military

Disclosure: The authors have nothing to disclose.
Psychology Service, VA Medical Center – Battle Creek, 5500 Armstrong Road, Battle Creek, MI 49037-7314, USA
* Corresponding author.
E-mail address: scott.driesenga@va.gov

Crit Care Nurs Clin N Am 27 (2015) 247–270
http://dx.doi.org/10.1016/j.cnc.2015.02.001   ccnursing.theclinics.com
0899-5885/15/$ – see front matter Published by Elsevier Inc.

Veteran population in a Veterans Affairs Medical Center (VAMC) setting, and to discuss implications for a general medical setting.

OVERVIEW OF POSTTRAUMATIC STRESS DISORDER AMONG VETERANS

Descriptions of a stress response syndrome to severe traumatic experiences have been documented since the beginning of time and have often been associated with warfare. The set of symptoms now typically identified as PTSD has previously been called shell shock, war neurosis, combat fatigue, battle stress, and gross stress reaction.[1] Following the terrorist attacks on September 11, 2001 and the subsequent wars in Iraq and Afghanistan, PTSD has become a common term within mainstream media and culture. The identification of a set of symptoms that were defined as a disorder in the psychiatric diagnostic manual nearly 35 years ago has generated a significant increase in research regarding PTSD.

It is well documented that PTSD has a significant negative impact on the physical, emotional, and mental health of individuals.[2–4] Furthermore, individuals with PTSD are more likely to be homeless, report increased marital instability and divorce, and in general, report reduced life satisfaction.[5] There is also a great deal of research and clinical experience that demonstrates the effectiveness of treatment of PTSD. The purpose of this article is to describe the salient features of PTSD, the assessment and treatment of PTSD with a special focus on the military Veteran population in a VAMC setting, and to discuss implications for a general medical setting.

DESCRIPTION OF POSTTRAUMATIC STRESS DISORDER

The American Psychiatric Association revised the PTSD diagnostic criteria in the latest edition of the Diagnostic and Statistical Manual of Mental Disorders (DSM-5), released in 2013.[6] PTSD can occur after experiencing or witnessing an event that involved actual or threatened death, serious injury, or sexual violence. The individual must have directly experienced the traumatic event, witnessed the event as it occurred to others, learned that the event occurred to a close family member or friend, or experienced repeated or extreme exposure to aversive details of the trauma event (not through electronic media or pictures). Common types of traumatic situations include combat, child abuse, physical and sexual assault, motor vehicle accidents, and natural disasters.

There are 4 main symptom clusters associated with a diagnosis of PTSD. These main symptom clusters include intrusive symptoms, avoidance, negative changes in thoughts and mood, and changes in arousal and reactivity. Specific symptoms are required in each of these 4 clusters to meet diagnostic criteria. (Please see DSM-5 criteria for PTSD for full description of symptoms within each cluster.) Additional criteria include duration of symptom disturbance of more than 1 month, significant distress or functional impairment related to the symptoms, and the determination that the symptoms are not due to physiologic effects of substance use or medical conditions. Furthermore, providers specify the presence or absence of dissociative symptoms and whether the onset is delayed (equal to or greater than 6 months' duration before symptom presentation).

PREVALENCE OF POSTTRAUMATIC STRESS DISORDER

The prevalence of exposure to trauma and resulting PTSD is relatively high in the general population (**Table 1**). The National Comorbidity Survey Replication (NCS-R) conducted interviews of a nationally representative sample of 9282 Americans aged

Table 1 Prevalence rates of posttraumatic stress disorder		
	Rates	
Population	Current	Lifetime
Vietnam Veterans	8.1%–15.2%	26.9%–30.9%
Persian Gulf Veterans	12.10%	11.2%–15.7%
OEF/OIF/OND Veterans	13.8%–15.8%	N/A
US general population	1.8%–5.2%	3.6%–9.7%

Abbreviations: N/A, not applicable; OEF, Operation Enduring Freedom; OIF, Operation Iraqi Freedom; OND, Operation New Dawn.

18 years and older.[7,8] PTSD was assessed among 5692 participants, using DSM-IV criteria. The NCS-R estimated the lifetime prevalence of PTSD among adult Americans to be 6.8%.[7] Past year prevalence of PTSD during the study period was estimated at 3.5%.[8] The lifetime prevalence of PTSD among men was 3.6% and among women was 9.7%. Current past year prevalence was 1.8% among men and 5.2% among women. The National Epidemiologic Survey on Alcohol and Related Conditions, a national survey conducted from 2004 to 2005, found a lifetime prevalence of PTSD of 7.3%.[9]

PREVALENCE OF POSTTRAUMATIC STRESS DISORDER IN VETERANS
Vietnam Veterans

The National Vietnam Veterans Readjustment Study conducted interviews of 3016 American Veterans conducted from 1986 to 1988.[10] These Veterans were selected to provide a representative sample of those who served in the Armed Forces during the Vietnam era. The estimated lifetime prevalence of PTSD among these Veterans was 30.9% for men and 26.9% for women. Of Vietnam theater Veterans, 15.2% of men and 8.1% of women were diagnosed with PTSD at the time the study was conducted.

Persian Gulf War Veterans

Kang and others[11,12] conducted a study to estimate the prevalence of PTSD in a population-based sample of 11,441 Gulf War Veterans from 1995 to 1997. PTSD was assessed using the PTSD Checklist (PCL) rather than interviews. The PCL is a self-report measure that assesses PTSD symptoms and symptom severity. In the study by Kang and colleagues,[12] those participants scoring 50 or higher were considered to have met criteria for PTSD. The prevalence of current PTSD in this sample of Gulf War Veterans was 12.1%. The lifetime prevalence was 11.2% for men and 15.7% for women. Furthermore, the authors estimated the prevalence of PTSD among the total Gulf War Veteran population to be 10.1%.

Operation Enduring Freedom/Operation Iraqi Freedom

In 2008, the RAND Corporation, Center for Military Health Policy Research, published a study that examined the prevalence of PTSD among service members who had been deployed for Operation Enduring Freedom or Operation Iraqi Freedom (OEF/OIF, wars in Afghanistan and Iraq, respectively).[13] Among the 1938 participants, the prevalence of current PTSD was 13.8%. More recently, results from the National Health Study for a New Generation of US Veterans were published.[14] The National Health Study for a New Generation of US Veterans is a longitudinal study of 60,000 Veterans, including

30,000 who served in Afghanistan and Iraq. The authors found that 15.8% of OEF/OIF deployed Veterans screened positive for PTSD using the PCL as the screening measure.

RISK FACTORS AND PROTECTIVE FACTORS FOR THE DEVELOPMENT OF POSTTRAUMATIC STRESS DISORDER

Most people (more than half) will experience at least one traumatizing event in their lifetime.[15] Most individuals who experience a trauma will naturally recover. These individuals do not develop a mental health disorder. However, there is a group of individuals who experience trauma who do develop mental health difficulties, one of which is PTSD. The reasons for this are not completely clear, but certainly are related to risk and protective factors as well as other obstacles to this natural recovery process. If the obstacles can be determined and/or removed, the process of recovery can be restarted. Within a Veteran population, severity of trauma, in terms of both the type of trauma experienced and the amount of trauma exposure, is the best predictor of the likelihood of developing PTSD, as well as the severity of PTSD symptoms.[13] Gender is also a risk factor. Although men are more likely to experience a traumatic event, women are more likely to experience the kind of traumatic event that can lead to PTSD, such as interpersonal violence and sexual assault. Additional risk factors for Veterans include having experienced traumatic experiences before serving in the military, the absence of a positive social support system, experiencing significant stress after the traumatic event, and engaging in significant avoidance behaviors.[16]

Conversely, there is evidence that protective factors exist that can protect an individual from developing PTSD. These protective factors may include seeking out social support and/or joining a support group after the traumatic event, having positive coping strategies, having a positive perspective on one's response to the trauma, and having an altruistic attitude toward others.[17] Hardiness as a personality trait (ie, having a realistic sense of control, being open to change, feeling that life is meaningful) also seems to be a protective factor.[18]

TREATMENT UTILIZATION AND BARRIERS

One encouraging finding when examining treatment utilization among Veterans with PTSD is that a greater numbers of Veterans are accessing PTSD-related services. In fact, Shiner and colleagues[19] found that nearly 58% of OEF/OIF Veterans have received some form of PTSD-related care. However, when examining the quality of care received, results are less promising. Research has demonstrated that only between 10% and 33% of Veterans with a diagnosis of PTSD receive "minimally adequate treatment."[20–22] As defined by Spoont and colleagues,[22] minimally adequate treatment entails a 4-month course of psychotropic medication and/or 8 psychotherapy sessions. Given that this criterion does not indicate the quality of treatment received (ie, provision of evidence-based treatments), these estimates may actually be the best case approximation of adequate treatment provision. For these reasons, it is important to examine specific barriers that may interfere with treatment engagement, whether this is initiation of treatment or a follow through with an adequate course of treatment of PTSD.

Stecker and colleagues[23] examined barriers to treatment engagement among 143 military personnel who screened positive for PTSD but had not yet engaged in mental health treatment. Barriers fell within 4 categories from most to least impactful: concerns regarding treatment, emotional readiness, stigma, and logistical problems. Primary concerns regarding treatment included not wanting to take medication for mental health difficulties, displeasure with group therapy options, and fear that providers will not understand the individual. Beliefs that treatment is not needed, that there is not a problem, that the individual is not ready, and that current coping skills, typically substance use, are sufficient to deal with symptoms were cited by participants related to emotional readiness. Stigma was examined from both the individual and the societal level. Self-stigma related to negative self-appraisals of seeking treatment (eg, sign of weakness). Fear of negative consequences related to security clearance, deployments, and future work was common and also related to beliefs regarding societal stigma (ie, belief that others will see the individual as crazy or unstable). Finally, logistical problems, such as lack of time for treatment, distance to the nearest facility, and family concerns, were cited as significant barriers to treatment engagement.

Another study examining barriers to treatment among Veterans Affairs (VA) service users who received a recent diagnosis of PTSD also found that negative beliefs regarding treatment were a significant barrier to mental health treatment engagement.[24] In addition, the current study examined the impact of social norms and messages from family, friends, other Veterans, and providers regarding treatment engagement. Findings demonstrated that Veterans whose social network did not encourage treatment seeking were less likely to engage in follow-up mental health care. Clearly, social encouragement or the lack thereof can either function as a facilitator or a barrier to treatment.

Sayer and her colleagues[25] examined barriers to treatment among 44 Veterans who were seeking disability compensation for PTSD. Although the current results are similar to previous studies regarding barriers (eg, negative treatment-related beliefs, access barriers, logistical barriers), 2 additional barriers were identified. Sayer and colleagues found that lack of knowledge and previous experiences with invalidation also significantly contributed to treatment hesitation. Lack of knowledge regarding PTSD, treatments for PTSD, and types of trauma that can contribute to the development of PTSD were reported. In addition, previous experience with invalidation of experiences and difficulties from the military and society were cited. Many Veterans identified negative experiences during homecoming, social norms against help-seeking, and a military culture that promoted silence after a trauma as significant reasons to refrain from seeking treatment. In the current study, reported barriers were also examined by dividing the participants into 2 groups, those currently receiving mental health treatment for PTSD and those not engaged in treatment. Interestingly, the results demonstrated that these 2 groups identified many of the same beliefs regarding barriers to treatment. Clearly, the barriers identified do not tell the whole story regarding why some Veterans decide not to seek treatment but are a starting point for further discussion and intervention.

Most studies examining barriers to engaging in treatment have primarily focused on beliefs, stigma, logistical issues, and social support[23–25] as primary predictors of treatment engagement. Nevertheless, other factors have demonstrated a significant relationship with a lack of engagement in mental health treatment. Age, service-connection status, and receipt of a diagnosis of PTSD in a non-mental health clinic have been shown to impact treatment initiation.[20,24] Older Veterans (age 30 and greater), those with a service-connected disability, and those who were diagnosed with PTSD in a non-mental health clinic (eg, primary care clinic) were less likely to engage in treatment. Even among this group of Veterans, those who chose to initially engage in treatment were less likely to complete an adequate course of treatment than those who were younger, those who were nonservice connected, and those who received their diagnosis in a mental health clinic.

ASSESSMENT OF POSTTRAUMATIC STRESS DISORDER

Completing a thorough assessment is critical in meeting the clinical needs of individuals with PTSD. Meeting standards for provision of evidence-based care involves making accurate diagnostic judgments and case conceptualizations that serve to guide treatment. It also requires the ongoing monitoring of treatment to inform and modify as necessary.[26] A comprehensive assessment will improve decision-making by providing information about the individual's current symptoms, comorbid conditions, coping mechanisms, and personality functioning. Furthermore, assessment can provide valuable information regarding an accurate diagnoses of PTSD as there may be several issues, such as secondary gain, that can impact an individuals presentation. Finally, ongoing assessment will assist with program evaluation and measurement of outcomes of treatment.

A thorough psychosocial assessment is critical, including a complete history, mental status assessment, and risk assessment. In addition to the psychosocial interview, there are many instruments available to assess for PTSD. There are several important considerations in the selection of the appropriate instruments to use in completing an assessment for PTSD. These considerations include setting of the assessment, reading level of the individual being assessed, time required to complete the assessment, costs of the measures, scope of the assessment, and psychometrics of the measures.

There are many screening tools that can be used to assist in identifying individuals who may have PTSD. The 4-item Primary Care PTSD Screen (PC-PTSD)[27] is one such instrument (**Box 1**). Generally, if an individual answers yes to 3 of the 4 items, it is considered a positive screen. Individuals who screen positive should then be assessed more thoroughly for PTSD using structured interviews and other instruments. The PC-PTSD is primarily designed to be used in primary care and other medical settings.

There are a multitude of self-report measures of PTSD available. The most widely used measure within the VA setting is the PCL. With the publication of DSM-5, the PCL[11] was updated to the PCL-5.[28] The PCL-5 is a 20-item instrument that assesses the 20 symptoms of PTSD in DSM-5. The PCL is effective as a screening tool for

---

Box 1
Primary care posttraumatic stress disorder screen

In your life, have you ever had any experience that was so frightening, horrible, or upsetting that, in the past month, you

1. Have had nightmares about it or thought about it when you did not want to?

   YES/NO

2. Tried hard not to think about it or went out of your way to avoid situations that reminded you of it?

   YES/NO

3. Were constantly on guard, watchful, or easily startled?

   YES/NO

4. Felt numb or detached from others, activities, or your surroundings?

   YES/NO

From Prins A, Ouimette P, Kimerling R, et al. The primary care PTSD screen (PC-PTSD): development and operating characteristics. Primary Care Psychia 2004;9:10.

PTSD, for making a provisional diagnosis of PTSD, and for monitoring symptom change during treatment. Other self-report measures with strong psychometric support include but are not limited to the Mississippi Scale for Combat-Related PTSD,[29] Impact of Event Scale–Revised,[30] Posttraumatic Diagnostic Scale,[31] and PTSD Symptom Scale–Self-Report Version.[32]

The Clinician-Administered PTSD Scale for DSM-5[33] is broadly recognized as the gold standard in PTSD assessment. This assessment is a 30-item structured interview that thoroughly assesses the 20 DSM-5 PTSD symptoms with questions that identify the onset, duration, and severity of symptoms as well as evaluates the distress of the interviewee, impact of symptoms on functioning, and improvement of symptoms over time with respect to a specified index trauma. This interview typically takes 45 to 60 minutes to complete. Additional adult interviews are available as well (eg, the PTSD Symptom Scale–Interview and Structured Clinical Interview for the DSM-IV Axis I Disorders).[32,34]

In addition to measures specific to the assessment for PTSD, it is beneficial to assess general personality functioning as well as comorbidities. The Minnesota Multiphasic Personality Inventory-2 (MMPI-2) is an instrument that has been extensively researched and used.[35] The MMPI-2 is an instrument with several validity scales that are useful in identifying the individuals' test-taking approach (eg, defensiveness, tendency toward over reporting and underreporting). The MMPI-2 is also beneficial in identifying an individual's personality functioning, general adjustment, and presence of psychopathology. For reference, the psychological assessment battery used by the Battle Creek VAMC PTSD Residential Program, measuring several domains, is listed in **Table 2**. Certainly, as described above, there are many well-validated measures that can be used to assess for PTSD and comorbid difficulties and diagnoses; however, the current list may be used as a resource and to illustrate the complexity

Table 2
Posttraumatic stress disorder–Residential Rehabilitation Treatment Program assessment battery

Instrument	Domain	Reference
ASI-III	Anxiety	36
BAM	Substance abuse	37
BASIS-24	Functioning	38
BDI-II	Depression	39
CBAS	Avoidance	40
CFS	Cognitive flexibility	41
FFMQ	Mindfulness	42
ISI	Insomnia	43
LEC	Traumatic life events	44
MMPI-II	Personality functioning	35,45
PCL-C, PCL-5	PTSD	11,28
PTGI-SF	Posttraumatic growth	46

Abbreviations: ASI-III, Anxiety Sensitivity Index–Third Edition; BAM, Brief Addiction Monitor; BASIS-24, Behavior and Symptom Identification Scale; BDI-II, Beck Depression Inventory–Second Edition; CBAS, Cognitive Behavioral Avoidance Scale; CFS, Cognitive Flexibility Scale; FFMQ, Five Facet Mindfulness Questionnaire; ISI, Insomnia Severity Index; LEC, Life Events Checklist; PCL-C, Posttraumatic Checklist–Civilian Version; PTGI-SF, Posttraumatic Growth Inventory–Short Form.
Data from Refs.[11,28,35–46]

of symptoms, difficulties, and strengths that can be assessed with a thorough assessment battery.

TREATMENT OF POSTTRAUMATIC STRESS DISORDER

Given the wealth of information regarding treatments for PTSD and the need to disseminate treatment recommendations to frontline staff, several agencies have developed practice guidelines. The International Society for Traumatic Stress Studies[47] and the Department of Veterans Affairs and Department of Defense[48] published clinical practice guidelines for the management of PTSD, identifying and categorizing treatments based on the results of available research. In addition, recommendations are offered regarding the progression and course of treatment to help clinicians maximally proceed with treatment. The following information is a summary of these findings with the addition of more recent published research.

There are several treatments available that have proven to be highly effective in the treatment of PTSD. Treatment may begin with education about common reactions to trauma and the key characteristics of PTSD. A coping skills approach that focuses on assisting the individual in identifying skills deficits and learning more adaptive coping strategies can be quite helpful. Many individuals with PTSD experience significant anxiety, anger, and irritability and have a difficult time managing their emotions. Developing anxiety and anger management skills and distress tolerance skills can be very beneficial. Often, this initial phase of treatment includes relaxation training, mindfulness, identifying and coping with triggers, assertiveness skills, anxiety and anger management skills training, behavioral activation (BA), sleep enhancement/hygiene, motivational interviewing, and distress tolerance skills training.

PSYCHOLOGICAL TREATMENTS FOR POSTTRAUMATIC STRESS DISORDER WITH STRONG EVIDENCE FOR EFFECTIVENESS

Two of the most effective treatments available for PTSD are prolonged exposure (PE)[49] and cognitive processing therapy (CPT).[50] Both PE and CPT are considered cognitive behavioral treatments, which emphasize the important role of one's thoughts, emotions, and behaviors. Cognitive behavioral treatments for PTSD often include several components, including psychoeducation, cognitive restructuring, exposure, and anxiety management elements.

PE is an 8- to 15-session treatment for PTSD that includes psychoeducation, relaxation/breathing retraining, and exposure.[49] During the first sessions of treatment, individuals are provided psychoeducation about common reactions to trauma, factors that maintain PTSD, the components of PE, the rationale for these components, and goals of treatment. Breathing retraining is a coping skill that individuals can use to help dampen physiologic arousal. It is essentially a quick tool that the clinician can teach the individual so that they have something to help them cope with their anxiety until exposure begins and starts to have an effect on functioning. Exposure, the process of repeatedly and systematically facing anxiety-provoking memories and situations until habituation occurs, is conducted in 2 forms: in vivo exposure and imaginal exposure. In vivo exposure involves confronting avoided situations that remind the individual of the trauma or cause the individual significant anxiety. A hierarchy of avoided/anxiety-producing situations is created and rated using a subjective unit of distress (SUDS) scale. SUDS ratings are used to enable the Veteran to quickly quantify how anxious they are at any given moment. Ratings range from 0 (no anxiety) to 100 (the most anxiety a person has experienced or can imagine experiencing). Individuals are then directed to face these situations in a structured manner, starting with situations with lower SUDS ratings and over time move up to situations that elicit higher SUDS ratings. Imaginal exposure involves having the individual revisit the trauma by recounting the trauma while imagining it. The specific traumatic situation selected, the index trauma, is retold several times in the session and is recorded. The individual is instructed to then listen to the recordings between sessions. Completion of treatment occurs when the individual reports that the identified trauma memory no longer causes them emotional distress and they are able to face previously avoided situations with minimal anxiety. Exposure allows individuals to learn that their anxiety will decrease (habituation) and that they can handle their anxiety, as well as gaining a new perspective on the trauma and increased confidence and competency. Results of studies on the impact of PE among Veterans have shown significant decreases in symptoms of PTSD as well as depression (eg,[51,52]).

CPT is a cognitive behavioral treatment that involves psychoeducation, cognitive restructuring, and written impact statements and trauma accounts.[50] Individuals are provided psychoeducation on the symptoms of PTSD, the process of recovery from trauma, the flight-fight-freeze response, the role of avoidance, a cognitive explanation of the formation of beliefs, and natural versus manufactured emotions. In addition, the concept of "stuck points" is introduced, those maladaptive, imbalanced thoughts that keep the individual stuck in maladaptive patterns of thinking and behaving and that impede the recovery process. Impact statements address how the trauma influenced the life of the individual in various ways (eg, beliefs about themselves, others, and the world) and their perceived meaning of the event and help the individual begin to identify their stuck points. Individuals are asked to write at least 2 trauma narratives during the course of treatment; this serves to help the individual express emotions about the trauma, put the trauma into a fuller context, and think about it in a more balanced way. During the second half of treatment, individuals are asked to challenge stuck points related to common themes such as safety, trust, power and control, esteem, and intimacy. Finally, individuals complete a second impact statement at the conclusion of treatment, which enables them to look at how the meaning of the event and their beliefs have changed over the course of treatment. Several researchers have examined the impact of CPT among Veterans with PTSD (eg,[53,54]) with significant positive findings related to reductions in symptoms of PTSD.

In addition to the cognitive behavioral treatments described above, there is also research support for eye movement desensitization and reprocessing (EMDR).[55] EMDR is an intervention that involves having the participant move their eyes back and forth (or engage in some other alternating activity such as tapping one hand then the other) while imagining the trauma. EMDR combines elements of exposure and cognitive behavioral treatment with the addition of eye movements. The eye movements are reported to enhance the elicitation of emotions while also seeming to make the traumatic recollection less vivid. EMDR also involves having the individual identify a more positive belief about the trauma and attempts to "install" that belief during the eye movements.

Stress inoculation training (SIT)[56] is a set of skills for managing anxiety and stress that has been found to be effective for individuals with PTSD.[57] SIT involves educating the client about stress and assists the client in developing stress management skills to "inoculate" the individual from future stress. SIT includes a conceptualization phase, a skills acquisition and rehearsal phase, and an application and follow-through phase. Typical skills included in SIT are emotional self-regulation, relaxation training, breathing retraining, assertiveness, positive thinking and self-talk, and thought stopping. When used with individuals with PTSD, SIT often includes an exposure component as well as a cognitive restructuring component. Therapeutic techniques, such as modeling, role playing, in vivo exposures, imagery, and behavioral rehearsal, are typically incorporated into SIT.

PSYCHOLOGICAL TREATMENTS FOR POSTTRAUMATIC STRESS DISORDER WITH SOME EVIDENCE FOR EFFECTIVENESS

Although originally developed for the treatment of depression, BA has shown promise in the treatment of PTSD as well.[58] BA is a brief, structured approach that targets avoidance and promotes engagement in pleasant and/or meaningful activities. Individuals with PTSD generally avoid people, places, and activities that may remind them of the trauma. This avoidance leads to social isolation and reduces the opportunities that the individual has to engage in rewarding activities. In BA, individuals are educated about PTSD and the relationship between avoidance and PTSD. They learn to identify avoidance behaviors, set goals, and engage in meaningful activities. Daily activity and mood charts are typically used and individuals are trained to identify triggers to anxiety, their responses to the triggers, and consequences of their responses.

Seeking Safety (SS)[59] is designed for persons with comorbid PTSD and substance use difficulties. SS is a presented-focused, flexible coping skills approach to treatment offering 25 modules that present adaptive coping skills. Providers can select from the skills modules depending on the needs of the individual. SS has 5 key principles:

1. Safety (in relationships, thinking, emotions, and behaviors)
2. Integrated treatment (SS assumes that an integrated approach to the treatment of PTSD and substance abuse is essential)
3. Ideals (to counteract the loss of ideals experienced with both PTSD and substance use)
4. Four content areas (cognitive, behavioral, interpersonal, and case management)
5. Focus on the provider (importance of self-care, managing one's own reactions in treatment).

Several studies have examined the use of SS among Veterans with PTSD and concurrent substance use difficulties. For example, Boden and colleagues[60] found that SS resulted in greater reductions in substance use as compared with treatment as usual.

Acceptance and commitment therapy (ACT) helps individuals develop more psychological flexibility.[61] Six core processes are used in ACT to promote change: acceptance, cognitive fusion, being present, self as context, values, and committed action. Rather than changing the content of dysfunctional thoughts and emotions, ACT suggests that individuals change their relationship to these internal events. ACT emphasizes strategies to facilitate a value-driven life. Treatment targets experiential avoidance to facilitate experiential willingness. Case studies have suggested ACT has benefit in the treatment of individuals with PTSD.[62,63]

There has also been limited support demonstrated for complementary and alternative medicine (CAM) approaches, such as meditation, acupuncture, yoga, and relaxation. Despite limited research support, a recent survey of all VA-specialized PTSD treatment programs found that 96% reported that they offered CAM approaches.[64] Of note, practice guidelines recommend CAM approaches for those Veterans who refuse trauma-focused treatments.[48]

PSYCHOLOGICAL TREATMENTS FOR SPECIFIC ISSUES RELATED TO POSTTRAUMATIC STRESS DISORDER

Sleep difficulties are a very common problem for individuals with PTSD, who often have difficulties falling asleep, staying asleep, or getting a restful night of sleep.

Cognitive Behavioral Therapy for Insomnia (CBT-I)[65] aims to change sleep patterns and factors associated with falling and staying asleep. Clients are provided extensive education about sleep cycles, sleep habits and behaviors, and the impact of thoughts and worries. They are given a series of sleep assessments, assigned a sleep diary, and given assignments to help change sleep patterns. Lifestyle patterns that prohibit one from falling or staying asleep are explored and remediated. The following methods may be used:

- Stimulus control therapy
- Sleep restriction
- Sleep hygiene
- Sleep environment improvement
- Relaxation training

Imagery rehearsal therapy[66] or exposure, relaxation, and rescripting therapy,[67] a nightmare rescripting approach using psychoeducation, and imagery rescripting, can be used in combination with CBT-I for those individuals with recurring nightmares.[68]

As noted previously, social support is a protective factor related to the development and maintenance of PTSD. Integrative behavioral couple therapy (IBCT)[69] promotes acceptance and change and consists of 2 phases, the evaluation phase and the treatment phase. This treatment incorporates the 2 goals of acceptance and change as positive outcomes for couples undergoing the treatment. Couples who successfully complete treatment often show a greater emotional acceptance of each other. IBCT consists of 2 phases, an evaluation/feedback phase and an active treatment phase developed from the findings in the evaluation phase. Of note, a review of the literature indicated that although couples' therapy can often help with relationship satisfaction, it does not typically result in a reduction in symptoms of PTSD.[48]

TECHNOLOGY AND POSTTRAUMATIC STRESS DISORDER TREATMENT

Virtual reality treatment (VRT) consists of custom virtual environments that have been carefully designed to support exposure therapy of anxiety disorders. The treatment involves exposing the person with PTSD to a virtual environment that contains the feared situation, instead of taking the patient into the actual environment or having the patient imagine the traumatic situation. A systematic review of VRT studies for the treatment of PTSD demonstrated significantly greater decreases in PTSD symptoms compared with wait-list control.[70] Although these results are promising, further examination found VRT to be no more effective than traditional exposure therapy for PTSD. Therefore, although the use of VRT presents a novel approach to the treatment of PTSD, the cost of this technology may not be justified given the equivalent effectiveness of traditional exposure therapy.

Although not a treatment in itself, mobile applications (apps) are increasingly being used to support treatments and increase use of treatment skills outside the therapy office. Applications, such as the PTSD Coach, PE Coach, and CPT Coach, developed jointly by the Department of Veterans Affairs and Department of Defense, provide treatment support and resources that are easily accessible to Veterans and military personnel. The hope is that these devices will increase treatment compliance, adherence, and convenience.[71] One study completed by Kuhn and colleagues[72] examined the use of the PTSD Coach. Results demonstrated that the Veterans who participated in the study were moderately to extremely satisfied with the app and found the content to be moderately to very helpful in managing symptoms. Of note, respondents particularly liked the discretion/privacy the app allowed.

PSYCHOPHARMACOLOGIC INTERVENTIONS

As PTSD varies in severity, and it responds well to EBTs, medication is not essential for everybody. Still, given the robust response to medication,[48] the threshold to make a referral to a primary care provider (PCP) or psychiatrist should be low. If a patient is a danger to themselves or others, but not severe enough to warrant hospitalization, or if there are serious psychiatric comorbidities, referral should preferably be to a psychiatrist, as opposed to a PCP. Referral should be considered when there is difficulty coping with everyday stress, difficulty functioning at home or at work, irritability or other symptoms actively damaging the person's relationships, or a patient preference to consider medication as part of their treatment program.

Psychopharmacologic Interventions with Strong Research Support

Many PTSD symptoms respond quite well to appropriate medication. The group of first-line medications can improve symptoms in all 4 of the PTSD symptom clusters.[73] The medications considered first-line therapy for PTSD include the selective serotonin reuptake inhibitors (SSRIs; eg, paroxetine, sertraline) and the selective serotonin and norepinephrine reuptake inhibitor (SNRI; eg, venlafaxine).[48,73–75] Symptom reduction is generally observed within 2 to 4 weeks, although a reduction in anger and irritability has been seen within the first week.[76] In addition, nightmares and general sleep disturbance do respond over time to SSRIs and SNRIs.[48] Fortunately, these agents are also used in the treatment of some psychiatric disorders that are commonly comorbid with PTSD, such as depression, panic disorder, generalized anxiety disorder, social anxiety disorder, and obsessive-compulsive disorder. This fact is particularly fortunate, because it is often arguable whether a patient's symptoms should all be attributed to PTSD, or a second, separate diagnosis is warranted.

Psychopharmacologic Interventions with Moderate to Minimal Research Support

Although nightmares and general sleep disturbance do respond over time to SSRIs and SNRIs, some sleep difficulties are so problematic that they warrant quick intervention. Previous research demonstrates that nightmares respond well to the antihypertensive agent prazosin.[77] Agents for the treatment of insomnia include trazodone and hypnotics.[48]

The role of benzodiazepines in PTSD is controversial. Although it is well established that benzodiazepines are not helpful with the core symptoms of PTSD, they can be useful to help reduce anxiety and promote sleep.[73] Despite this, some experts argue that the problems of abuse, diversion, and dependence make these medications inadvisable.[48] There is consensus, however, that when they are prescribed, the goal should be the reduction of symptoms, not the complete elimination of symptoms. The lowest dose possible should be used and for the shortest duration of time. Non-habit-forming medications for insomnia should be attempted first (trazodone, low-dose Tricyclic antidepressants) before turning to benzodiazepines.

Prescribing Practices and Pharmacologic Special Issues

Certainly, the initial prescription provided to an individual is simply the first step in treatment. Follow-up visits are used to assess the effects of prescribed medications and side effects of medication and to make dosing adjustments as needed. Side effects are generally mild with first-line medications for PTSD and resolve over time.[48,75] Reassurance is appropriate in most cases. Patients should always be advised that, paradoxically, a new medication, or any increase or decrease in dose, can precipitate new-onset suicidal or aggressive thoughts in certain populations,[78] which should prompt an immediate evaluation by phone or in person. Clinicians may consider an increase in dose at follow-up visits if there is no response or a partial response.[48] If the maximum dose is reached and there is no response, the medication may be tapered and discontinued, and a second first-line medication initiated. If the maximum dose is reached with only a partial response, it is reasonable to either switch the patient to a different first-line agent or add an adjunctive medication to the first, such as a mood stabilizer, second antidepressant with a different mechanism of action, a second-generation antipsychotic medication, or others.

Special attention should be paid to the sexual side effects of the first-line medications, because these side effects often affect whether the Veteran agrees to begin and continue therapy.[79] It is recommended that a sexual history be taken at the initiation of therapy, with specific questions about the 3 phases of the sexual response: interest, arousal, and orgasm, because the medication can affect any and all phases. Clinicians may ask about frequency, because what patients consider "normal" varies significantly. Strategies used when patients report treatment-emergent sexual problems include counseling, holding the SSRI/SNRI dose on the day of intimacy, reducing frequency expectations, using sexual aids, dosage reduction, switching to another first-line medication, or adding a second medication to offset the problematic effect. For example, phosphodiesterase inhibitors in men (sildenafil, vardenafil, tadalafil) are commonly used. Other medications such as bupropion, buspirone, and yohimbine can also be prescribed.

Assessing and treating sleep difficulties are critical, because nightmares and/or poor sleep can hamper recovery. Physicians should take a thorough sleep history before beginning therapy. If there is any suspicion of sleep apnea or other medical causes, the patient should be referred for evaluation. Sleep apnea causes a dramatic increase in mortality, considerable morbidity from cardiac effects, as well as days spent in the hospital for adverse events.[80] Treatment of other sleep disorders should be guided by best practices for those conditions. (Please refer to the American Academy of Sleep Medicine for clinical standards.)

MANAGEMENT OF VETERANS WITH POSTTRAUMATIC STRESS DISORDER BY HEALTH CARE PROVIDERS

As noted previously, the prevalence of trauma in the general public is very high. Research suggests that about 60% of men and 50% women experience at least one trauma at some point in their lives.[81] There is a substantial amount of research that suggests that exposure to trauma and the development of PTSD may have a negative impact on physical health. For example, individuals with PTSD generally experience a high rate of comorbid medical disorders, such as arthritis, asthma, back pain, diabetes, eczema, kidney disease, lung disease, and ulcer.[82–85] It is critical for medical personnel to be aware of this. PTSD is highly prevalent in those who seek care in a primary care setting. Various studies have found that between 6% and 25% of individuals seen in a primary care setting are experiencing PTSD.[27,86,87] In one study, findings indicated that 11.5% of Veterans presenting to a primary care clinic were experiencing PTSD.[88] It has been estimated that about 60% of eligible Veterans do not receive their health care in a VA setting.[89] Rather, they receive their care in a private setting where their status as a Veteran may not be considered. In addition, patients with PTSD tend to have higher rates of health care utilization.[90,91] Several studies have shown that Veterans with PTSD are more likely to present to a primary care clinic than a mental health clinic. Likely, this is due to the stigma associated with mental health diagnoses and treatment, particularly strong in a Veteran population (eg,[23]).

Assessment and brief mental health treatment offered in a primary care setting can be a point of entry for individuals to pursue treatment in a mental health setting.

Greater collaboration between mental health professionals and primary care/specialty medical care professionals is essential. Primary care/medical care professionals can take several steps to improve the care provided to individuals with PTSD. First, it is recommended that mental health providers become members of the medical team. Mental health providers deliver invaluable services such as consultation, assessment, brief treatment, and referral for specialty mental health care. It is also important for PCPs to assess patients for Veteran status and to screen for PTSD in health care settings. The PC-PTSD has been specifically designed to be used in primary care/health care settings.[27]

A positive PTSD screen (at least 3 of the 4 items responded to affirmatively) (**Box 1**) is not enough information to definitively diagnose PTSD; however, it does indicate the need for further evaluation. It is recommended that individuals with a positive PC-PTSD be further assessed for PTSD. An assessment of whether the individual served in the military and/or served in a combat zone is critical to determining the presence of a traumatic event or events. Furthermore, a thorough risk assessment is indicated. Following a discussion of the results of the screen, the provider and patient can mutually determine whether it would be helpful to consult with a mental health professional, either one that is a member of the primary care team or a referral to a specialty mental health care professional. During this discussion, it is important for the PCP to provide information about common reactions to trauma, effective treatment options available to the individual, and the importance of maintaining a hopeful, recovery-oriented attitude. Given that providers in primary care clinics are often the first contact that Veterans have with VA providers, they typically serve as the gatekeepers of mental health treatment. Treatment initiation and engagement increase when providers in primary care clinics refer Veterans who screen positive for PTSD to mental health clinics for diagnosis and treatment[24,92] rather than retaining them in primary care clinics.

As noted above, it is highly beneficial for mental health professionals to be integral members of the medical team. VAMCs have been at the forefront of integrating mental health professionals into primary care teams. Studies suggest that brief psychological treatments can be effectively delivered in a primary care setting for many mental health conditions, including PTSD. A group of VAMC health care providers developed and piloted a brief intervention for PTSD for use in a primary care setting. The intervention, brief trauma treatment (BTT),[93] is 3 sessions in duration and each session is about 20 minutes in length, a treatment approach that fits well within a busy primary care clinic setting. One critical goal of BTT is to enhance the natural recovery process. BTT consists of 4 elements including education about common reactions to trauma, BA to pleasurable activities, motivational enhancement strategies, and patient-centered treatment planning. There were small but meaningful decreases in scores on self-report measures of mood and anxiety (although no drop in measures of PTSD symptoms). Most notable, about half of the participants were referred to and engaged in further treatment in a mental health setting, which is a significant improvement in mental health engagement as compared to rates found in previous studies.[19,94]

There are additional brief treatments for PTSD that have been offered in primary care settings. Jakupcak and colleagues[95] completed a pilot project exploring the use of BA and problem-solving therapy for PTSD and depression in Veterans who served in Iraq and Afghanistan. They found that the treatment, an 8-session protocol based on a BA model,[96] led to improvements in PTSD, depression, and quality of life. Additional treatment programs for PTSD designed for use in a primary care setting have been devised as well.[5]

SPECIAL ISSUES

There are many complicating factors that are important to consider when working with Veterans with a diagnosis of PTSD. First, co-occurring disorders are incredibly common and often complicate the clinical picture as well as the recommended course of treatment.[81,97–99] Most commonly, diagnoses of additional anxiety disorders, depressive disorders, and substance use disorders are assigned. Ginzburg and colleagues[98] completed a 20-year longitudinal study of Israeli War Veterans and found that co-occurrence of disorders tended to be the rule rather than the exception. Veterans were more likely to carry PTSD, anxiety disorder, and depressive disorder diagnoses concurrently than PTSD alone or a combination of PTSD and either an anxiety or a depressive disorder. In addition, the development of PTSD tended to precede the development of other disorders. Studies have shown that as many as 80% of individuals with PTSD have 3 or more current mental health problems and as many as 4 or more over the course of their lifetime. As many as half of the men with PTSD have co-occurring substance abuse problems.[81] Other disorders are also common among those with a diagnosis of PTSD, including personality disorders (most frequently, paranoid, avoidant, borderline, and obsessive-compulsive personality disorders)[97] and psychotic disorders.[100] For this reason, a thorough assessment of symptoms is needed to determine a clear diagnostic picture and provide solid treatment recommendations. For some disorders, concurrent treatment is recommended, as is the case for PTSD and substance use disorders (eg,[101,102]); whereas in other cases, treatment of the primary diagnosis may need to precede trauma-focused treatment of PTSD.

Traumatic brain injury (TBI) is also a significant concern, particularly with Veterans who served in Iraq and Afghanistan. TBI is considered one of the signature injuries of these wars. As a result of an increase in utilization of IEDs (improvised explosive devices) by enemy combatants, as well as improved protective gear used by American troops, service members have been more likely to survive physical injuries than in the past. Researchers have used varying methods, but overall, studies have found that 15% to 20% of individuals who served in Iraq and Afghanistan reported injuries that resulted in loss of consciousness. In one study, almost 44% of soldiers who reported loss of consciousness met PTSD criteria as well.[103] Most notably, long-term effects of TBI have been extensively studied among military personnel and Veterans.[104] Given that PTSD and TBI share many of the same difficulties (eg, reported difficulties with attention, memory, impulsivity/reckless behavior), differential diagnosis of these disorders is complicated. In addition, individuals with both diagnoses tend to experience more severe PTSD symptoms, self-awareness impairment, greater emotional reactivity, and reduced problem-solving efficiency (see[104] for a review of the literature). Preliminary studies examining the impact of CPT and PE on Veterans with PTSD and co-occurring TBI have shown promising results in reduction of symptoms.[105–107] It should be noted that most participants in these studies were diagnosed with mild or moderate TBI. Individuals with more severe TBI may benefit from further adjunctive treatment, such as those described in the above-mentioned studies by Chard and colleagues[105] and Walter and colleagues.[106] In addition, the VA developed the National Polytrauma System of Care to further address the unique challenges of this population and provide specialized care (see[108] for further information).

Several studies have examined the relationship between PTSD and suicide.[109–111] Results demonstrate that individuals with PTSD experience greater suicidal ideation, attempts, and completed suicide compared with individuals without a diagnosis. A co-occurring diagnosis of a depressive disorder further increases this risk. For this reason, assessment of risk and protective factors is critical. Risk factors can help identify those individuals who are more likely to consider suicide. Risk factors that may be relevant include history of trauma, physical health problems including untreated or undertreated pain, mental health problems, age, gender, access to weapons, previous suicide attempts, and lack of social support. Protective factors can include engagement in health care, positive social support, restricted access to weapons, hope for the future, and positive coping skills. Jacobs and Brewer[112] point out that direct questions about suicide are an essential tool in suicide assessment and need not be avoided. Every VA medical facility is required to have a suicide prevention program to respond to referrals and maintain a list of Veterans who are assessed to be at a high risk for suicide. This program allows these Veterans additional support as well as provides additional support and guidelines to providers. (For further information regarding assessing and addressing suicidal risk, please see the VA/DoD Clinical Practice Guidelines regarding the Assessment and Management of Patients at Risk for Suicide.[113])

Family concerns are a significant issue to consider when treating Veterans with PTSD, especially given the association between PTSD and negative family functioning.[114,115] PTSD has been associated with aggression/violent behavior, marital difficulties, partner distress, lower parental functioning, and increased behavioral issues among the children of Veterans with PTSD.[116] When examining how PTSD impacts the family, one study found that the method of coping with symptoms used by Veterans predicted family functioning. Specifically, an avoidant coping style was associated with greater family dysfunction as compared with an approach coping style.[114] Fortunately, there are several avenues of support for family, in the form of crisis services (eg, Veterans Crisis Line, National Domestic Violence Hotline, National Child Abuse Hotline, VA Caregiver Support Line) as well as supportive and preventative health services (eg, VA Caregiver Support, Coaching Into Care Program, National Resource Directory, Vet Center Combat Call Center). In addition, several studies have demonstrated positive effects of couples and family therapy.[48] (For further information on available family resources and treatments, please see the National Center for PTSD website.)

Women are a unique subset of the Veteran population with different needs and challenges. Previous research examining PTSD among women Veterans has shown that women tend to report a higher incidence of military sexual trauma (MST) than men and higher symptoms of PTSD.[117] Additional barriers to engagement in treatment are also present for women Veterans and range from low income, a lack of women-specific care, and the male-oriented nature of care at the VA.[117-120] For this reason, a women's Veterans program manager is identified and available at all sites who can help women Veterans receive needed service and advocate for the needs of women Veterans. In addition, gender-specific services are available for women Veterans, including Women's Stress Disorder Treatment Teams, specialized inpatient and residential programs for women, cohort treatment or separate wings for women, Women Veterans Comprehensive Health Centers, and Women Veterans Homelessness Programs. In addition, information on available resources and how to access local resources can be found on the National Center for PTSD website.

MST is a significant problem within the military. MST has been defined as "psychological trauma, which in the judgment of a VA mental health professional, resulted from a physical assault of a sexual nature, battery of a sexual nature, or sexual harassment which occurred while the Veteran was serving on active duty, active duty for training, or inactive duty training".[121] Although rates of MST are difficult to determine, often due to a lack of reporting, some studies have estimated that MST is experienced by upwards of 33% of women and 12% of men during their course of military service.[122,123] In addition, findings have shown that rates of PTSD are higher for individuals who have experienced MST (approximately 50%) than other types of trauma.[124] Preliminary studies have been completed with Veterans diagnosed with PTSD related to MST, indicating positive results of trauma-focused treatments such as CPT and PE.[125,126] Within the VA, providers are required to assess every Veteran for MST. Veterans who are positive for MST are eligible for free physical and mental health services related to their experience of MST. In addition, every VA site has a local MST coordinator who can help individuals connect with MST-related care and resources. Nationwide, there are MST programs available on an outpatient, residential, and inpatient basis. There are also designated facilities that offer gender-specific treatment based on Veteran preference. (For further information on available resources, please see the National Center for PTSD Web site.)

There is a growing recognition of Veterans' significant involvement with the justice system. Based on Bureau of Justice Statistics data,[127,128] on any given day, approximately 9.4% of the inmates in the country's prisons and jails are Veterans. Eighty-five percent of Veterans engaged in VAMC substance use disorder treatment programming reported at least one criminal charge.[129] It has been posited that one explanation for the high rates of justice involvement for Veterans may be a result of military training and the development of coping strategies that were adaptive in the military setting (aggressiveness, hypervigilance, arousal, instantaneous decision-making) but are maladaptive in civilian settings and may lead to difficulties such as aggressiveness, impulsiveness, and other behaviors that could result in legal issues and incarceration.[130] Veterans' involvement with the legal system has significant implications for treatment. Veterans involved with the justice system often present to treatment under court order, which can impact motivation for treatment. Special programs, such as "Veterans Court," have been developed. VAMCs have designated Veteran Justice Outreach workers who serve as liaisons between the legal system and the VAMC. These workers typically travel to jails and prisons, provide consultation, and identify Veterans who are incarcerated who may benefit from mental health treatment.

SUMMARY

PTSD is a common disorder among military personnel and Veterans that has a significant impact on the functioning and well-being of the individual. Several factors related to risk and barriers to treatment have been identified and are important to address when first meeting with Veterans in a primary care setting. Appropriate referral to mental health staff is recommended at the first sign that PTSD is a difficulty, because this has been shown to increase treatment engagement. Effective assessment and treatment of PTSD have been identified and are available. Psychometrically sound screening, self-report, interview, and objective measures are available and recommended for use in assessing for the presence of PTSD and co-occurring difficulties as well as differential diagnosis. Both psychological and psychopharmacologic interventions with particular evidence demonstrating their efficacy and effectiveness have been identified. Frontline treatments include cognitive behavioral treatments, such as PE and CPT, and/or the use of SSRIs. Finally, special consideration must be made regarding issues that are common and/or salient to this population, including co-occurring disorders, TBI, suicide, family issues, issues salient to women Veterans, MST, and legal issues.

REFERENCES

1. American Psychiatric Association. Diagnostic and statistical manual of mental disorders. Washington, DC: Author; 1952.

2. Wagner AW, Wolfe J, Rotnitsky A, et al. An investigation of the impact of post-traumatic stress disorder on physical health. J Trauma Stress 2000;13(1):41–55.

3. Zatzick DF, Marmar CR, Weiss DS, et al. Posttraumatic stress disorder and functioning and quality of life outcomes in a nationally representative sample of male Vietnam Veterans. Am J Psychiatry 1997;154(12):1690–5.

4. Kilpatrick DG, Resnick HS, Milanak ME, et al. National estimates of exposure to traumatic events and PTSD prevalence using DSM-IV and DSM-5 criteria. J Trauma Stress 2013;26:537–47.

5. Schnurr PP, Lunney CA, Bovin MJ, et al. Posttraumatic stress disorder and quality of life: extension of findings to Veterans of the wars in Iraq and Afghanistan. Clin Psychol Rev 2009;29:727–35.

6. American Psychiatric Association. Diagnostic and statistical manual of mental disorders. 5th edition. Washington, DC: American Psychiatric Association; 2013.

7. Kessler RC, Berglund P, Delmer O, et al. Lifetime prevalence and age-of-onset distributions of DSM-IV disorders in the National Comorbidity Survey Replication. Arch Gen Psychiatry 2005;62(6):593–602.

8. Kessler RC, Chiu WT, Demler O, et al. Prevalence, severity, and comorbidity of 12-month DSM-IV disorders in the National Comorbidity Survey Replication. Arch Gen Psychiatry 2005;62(6):617–27.

9. Roberts AL, Gilman SE, Breslau J, et al. Race/ethnic differences in exposure to traumatic events, development of post-traumatic stress disorder, and treatment-seeking for post-traumatic stress disorder in the United States. Psychol Med 2011;41(1):71–83.

10. Kulka RA, Schlenger WA, Fairbanks JA, et al. Trauma and the Vietnam War generation: report of findings from the National Vietnam Veterans Readjustment Study. New York: Brunner/Mazel; 1990.

11. Weathers F, Litz B, Herman D, et al. The PTSD checklist (PCL): reliability, validity, and diagnostic utility. San Antonio (TX): Annual Convention of the International Society for Traumatic Stress Studies; 1993.

12. Kang HK, Natelson BH, Mahan CM, et al. Post-traumatic stress disorder and chronic fatigue syndrome-like illness among Gulf War Veterans: a population-based survey of 30,000 Veterans. Am J Epidemiol 2003;157(2):141–8.

13. Tanielian T, Jaycox L, editors. Invisible wounds of war: psychological and cognitive injuries, their consequences, and services to assist recovery. Santa Monica (CA): RAND Corporation; 2008.

14. Dursa EK, Reinhard MJ, Barth SK, et al. Prevalence of a positive screen for PTSD among OEF/OIF and OEF/OIF-era Veterans in a large population-based cohort. J Trauma Stress 2014;27(5):542–9.

15. Spoont M, Arbisi P, Fu S, et al. Screening for post-traumatic stress disorder (PTSD) in primary care: a systematic review. Washington (DC): Department of Veterans Affairs; 2013.

16. Brewin CR, Andrews B, Valentine JD. Meta-analysis of risk factors for posttraumatic stress disorder in trauma-exposed adults. J Consult Clin Psychol 2000; 68(5):748–66.

17. Charney DS. Psychobiological mechanisms of resilience and vulnerability: implications for successful adaptation to extreme stress. Am J Psychiatry 2004; 161(2):195–216.

18. King LA, King DW, Fairbank JA, et al. Resilience-recovery factors in post-traumatic stress disorder among female and male Vietnam Veterans: hardiness, postwar social support, and additional stressful life events. J Pers Soc Psychol 1998;74(2):420–34.

19. Shiner B, Drake RE, Watts BV, et al. Access to VA services for returning Veterans with PTSD. Mil Med 2012;177(7):814–22.
20. Lu MW, Carlson KF, Duckart JP, et al. The effects of age on initiation of mental health treatment after positive PTSD screens among Veterans affairs primary care patients. Gen Hosp Psychiatry 2012;34(6):654–9.
21. Seal KH, Maguen S, Cohen B, et al. VA mental health services utilization in Iraq and Afghanistan Veterans in the first year of receiving new mental health diagnoses. J Trauma Stress 2010;23(1):5–16.
22. Spoont MR, Murdoch M, Hodges J, et al. Treatment receipt by Veterans after a PTSD diagnosis in PTSD, mental health, or general medical clinics. Psychiatr Serv 2010;61(1):58–63.
23. Stecker T, Shiner B, Watts BV, et al. Treatment-seeking barriers for Veterans of the Iraq and Afghanistan conflicts who screen positive for PTSD. Psychiatr Serv 2013;64(3):280–3.
24. Spoont MR, Nelson DB, Murdoch M, et al. Impact of treatment beliefs and social network encouragement on initiation of care by VA service users with PTSD. Psychiatr Serv 2014;65(5):654–62.
25. Sayer NA, Friedemann-Sanchez G, Spoont MR, et al. A qualitative study of determinants of PTSD treatment initiation in Veterans. Psychiatry 2009;72(3): 238–55.
26. American Psychological Association, Presidential Task Force on Evidence-Based Practice. Evidence-based practice in psychology. Am Psychol 2006; 61(4):271–85.
27. Prins A, Ouimette P, Kimerling R, et al. The primary care PTSD screen (PC-PTSD): development and operating characteristics. Primary Care Psychia 2003;9(1):9–14.
28. Weathers FW, Litz BT, Keane TM, et al. The PTSD checklist for DSM-5 (PCL-5). Washington (DC): National Center for PTSD; 2013. Available at: www.ptsd.va.gov. Accessed November 11, 2014.
29. Hyer L, Davis H, Boudewyns PA, et al. A short form of the Mississippi scale for combat-related PTSD. J Clin Psychol 1991;47(4):510–8.
30. Weiss DS, Marmar CR. The impact of event scale—revised. In: Wilson J, Keane TM, editors. Assessing psychological trauma and PTSD. New York: Guilford Press; 1997. p. 399–411.
31. Foa EB, Cashman L, Jaycox L, et al. The validation of a self-report measure of posttraumatic stress disorder: the posttraumatic diagnostic scale. Psychol Assess 1997;9(4):445–51.
32. Foa E, Riggs D, Dancu C, et al. Reliability and validity of a brief instrument for assessing post-traumatic stress disorder. J Trauma Stress 1993;6:459–74.
33. Weathers FW, Blake DD, Schnurr PP, et al. The clinician-administered PTSD scale for DSM-5 (CAPS-5). Washington (DC): National Center for PTSD; 2013. Available at: www.ptsd.va.gov. Accessed November 11, 2014.
34. First MB, Spitzer RL, Gibbon M, et al. Structured clinical interview for DSM-IV axis I disorders, clinician version (SCID-CV). Washington, DC: American Psychiatric Press, Inc; 1996.
35. Butcher JN, Dahlstrom WG, Graham JR, et al. The Minnesota multiphasic personality inventory-2 (MMPI-2) manual for administration and scoring. Minneapolis (MN): University of Minneapolis; 1989.
36. Taylor S, Zvolensky MJ, Cox BJ, et al. Robust dimensions of anxiety sensitivity: development and initial validation of the Anxiety Sensitivity Index-3. Psychol Assess 2007;19:176–88.

37. Cacciola JS, Alterman AI, DePhillippis D, et al. Development and initial evaluation of the Brief Addiction Monitor (BAM). J Subst Abuse Treat 2013;44:256–63.

38. Eisen SV, Norman SL, Belager AJ, et al. The revised behavior and symptom identification scale (BASIS-R): reliability and validity. Med Care 2004;42: 1230–41.

39. Beck AT, Steer RA, Carbin MG. Psychometric properties of the beck depression inventory: twenty-five years of evaluation. Clin Psychol Rev 1998;8:77–100.

40. Ottenbreit ND, Dobson KS. An examination of avoidance in the context of depression. Behav Res Ther 2004;42:293–313.

41. Martin MM, Rubin RB. A new measure of cognitive flexibility. Psychol Rep 1995; 76:623–6.

42. Baer RA, Smith GT, Hopkins J, et al. Using self-report assessment methods to explore facets of mindfulness. Assessment 2006;13(1):27–45.

43. Morin CM, Belleville G, Belanger L, et al. The Insomnia Severity Index: psychometric indicators to detect insomnia cases and evaluate treatment response. Sleep 2011;34:601–8.

44. Gray MJ, Litz BT, Hsu JL, et al. Psychometric properties of the life events checklist. Assessment 2004;11:330–41.

45. Glenn DM, Beckham JC, Sampson WS, et al. MMPI-2 profiles of gulf and Vietnam combat Veterans with chronic posttraumatic stress disorder. J Clin Psychol 2007;58:371–81.

46. Palmer GA, Graca JJ, Occhetti KE. Confirmatory factor analysis of the posttraumatic growth inventory in a Veteran sample with posttraumatic stress disorder. J Loss Trauma 2012;17:545–56.

47. Foa EB, Keane TM, Friedman MJ, et al. Effective treatments for PTSD: practice guidelines from the International Society for Traumatic Stress Studies. New York: Guilford Press; 2005.

48. Department of Veterans Affairs, Department of Defense. VA/DoD clinical practice guideline for the management of posttraumatic stress disorder. Washington, DC: Department of Veterans Affairs, Department of Defense; 2010.

49. Foa EB, Hembree EA, Rothbaum BO. Prolonged exposure therapy for PTSD: emotional processing of traumatic experiences. New York: Oxford University Press; 2007.

50. Resick PA, Monson CM, Chard KM. Cognitive processing therapy treatment manual: Veteran/military version. Boston: Veterans Administration; 2013.

51. Tuerk PW, Yoder M, Grubaugh A, et al. Prolonged exposure therapy for combat-related posttraumatic stress disorder: an examination of treatment effectiveness for Veterans of the wars in Afghanistan and Iraq. J Anxiety Disord 2011;25(3): 397–403.

52. Thorp SR, Stein MB, Jeste DV, et al. Prolonged exposure therapy for older Veterans with posttraumatic stress disorder: a pilot study. Am J Geriatr Psychiatry 2012;20(3):276–80.

53. Karlin BE, Ruzek JI, Chard KM, et al. Dissemination of evidence-based psychological treatments for posttraumatic stress disorder in the Veterans Health Administration. J Trauma Stress 2010;23(6):663–73.

54. Chard KM, Schumm JA, Owens GP, et al. A comparison of OEF and OIF Veterans and Vietnam Veterans receiving cognitive processing therapy. J Trauma Stress 2010;23(1):25–32.

55. Shapiro F. Eye movement desensitization and reprocessing. 2nd edition. New York: The Guilford Press; 2001.

56. Meichenbaum D. Stress inoculation training. New York: Pergamon Press; 1985.

57. Hembree EA, Foa EB. Posttraumatic stress disorder: psychological factors and psychosocial interventions. J Clin Psychiatry 2000;61(Suppl 7):33–9.
58. Jakupcak M, Roberts LJ, Martell C, et al. A pilot study of behavioral activation for Veterans with posttraumatic stress disorder. J Trauma Stress 2006;19(3): 387–91.
59. Najavits LM. Seeking safety: a treatment manual for PTSD and substance abuse. New York: Guilford Press; 2002.
60. Boden MT, Kimerling RE, Jacobs-Lentz J, et al. Seeking safety treatment for male Veterans with a substance use disorder and post-traumatic stress disorder symptomatology. Addiction 2012;107(3):578–86.
61. Hayes SC, Strosahl KD, Wilson KG. Acceptance and commitment therapy: the process and practice of mindful change. 2nd edition. New York: Guilford Press; 2011.
62. Batten SV, Hayes SC. Acceptance and commitment therapy in the treatment of comorbid substance abuse and post-traumatic stress disorder: a case study. Clin Case Stud 2005;4:246–62.
63. Orsillo SM, Batten SV. Acceptance and commitment therapy in the treatment of posttraumatic stress disorder. Behav Modif 2008;29:95–129.
64. Libby DJ, Pilver CE, Desai R. Complementary and alternative medicine in VA specialized PTSD treatment programs. Psychiatr Serv 2012b;63:1134–6.
65. Jacobs GD, Pace-Schott EF, Stickgold R, et al. Cognitive behavior therapy and pharmacotherapy for insomnia: a randomized controlled trial and direct comparison. Arch Intern Med 2004;164:1888–96.
66. Cook JM, Thompson R, Harb GC, et al. Cognitive–behavioral treatment for posttraumatic nightmares: an investigation of predictors of dropout and outcome. Psychol Trauma 2013;5(6):545–53.
67. Davis JL, Wright DC. Exposure, relaxation, and rescripting treatment for trauma-related nightmares. J Trauma Dissociation 2006;7(1):5–18.
68. Margolies SO, Rybarczyk B, Vrana SR, et al. Efficacy of a cognitive-behavioral treatment for insomnia and nightmares in Afghanistan and Iraq Veterans with PTSD. J Clin Psychol 2013;69(10):1026–42.
69. Christensen A, Jacobson NS, Babcock JC. Integrative behavioral couples therapy. In: Jacobson NS, Gurman AS, editors. Clinical handbook for couples therapy. New York: Guildford; 1995. p. 31–64.
70. Gonçalves R, Pedrozo AL, Coutinho ESF, et al. Efficacy of virtual reality exposure therapy in the treatment of PTSD: a systematic review. PLoS One 2012;7(12).
71. Reger GM, Hoffman J, Riggs D, et al. The "PE coach" smartphone application: an innovative approach to improving implementation, fidelity, and homework adherence during prolonged exposure. Psychol Serv 2013;10(3):342–9.
72. Kuhn E, Greene C, Hoffman J, et al. Preliminary evaluation of PTSD Coach, a smartphone app for post-traumatic stress symptoms. Mil Med 2014;179(1):12–8.
73. American Psychiatric Association. Practice guideline for the treatment of patients with acute stress disorder and posttraumatic stress disorder. 2010. Available at: http://psychiatryonline.org/pb/assets/raw/sitewide/practice_guidelines/guidelines/acutestressdisorderptsd.pdf. Accessed February 1, 2012.
74. Ipser JC, Stein DJ. Evidence-based pharmacotherapy of post-traumatic stress disorder (PTSD). Int J Neuropsychopharmacol 2012;15(6):825–40.
75. Davidson J, Baldwin D, Stein DJ. Treatment of posttraumatic stress disorder with venlafaxine extended release: a 6-month randomized controlled trial. Arch Gen Psychiatry 2006;63(10):1158–65.

76. Davidson JR, Landerman LR, Farfel GM, et al. Characterizing the effects of sertraline in post-traumatic stress disorder. Psychol Med 2002;32(4):661–70.
77. Kung S, Espinel Z, Lapid MI. Treatment of nightmares with prazosin: a systematic review. Mayo Clin Proc 2012;87(9):890–900.
78. Barbui C, Esposito E, Cipriani A. Selective serotonin reuptake inhibitors and risk of suicide: a systematic review of observational studies. Can Med Assoc J 2009; 180(3):291–7.
79. Gitlin M. Sexual dysfunction with psychotropic drugs. Expert Opin Pharmacother 2003;4(12):2259–69.
80. Fonseca MI, Pereira T, Caseiro P. Death and disability in patients with sleep apnea: a meta-analysis. Arq Bras Cardiol 2015;104(1):58–66.
81. Kessler RC, Sonnega A, Bromet E, et al. Posttraumatic stress disorder in the National Comorbidity Study. Arch Gen Psychiatry 1995;52:1048–60.
82. Spiro A, Hankins CS, Mansell D, et al. Posttraumatic stress disorder and health status: the Veterans Health Study. J Ambul Care Manage 2006;29(1): 71–86.
83. Schnurr PP, Spiro A, Paris AH. Physician-diagnosed medical disorders in relation to PTSD symptoms in older male military Veterans. Health Psychol 2000; 19(1):91–7.
84. Schnurr PP, Friedman MJ, Sengupta A, et al. PTSD and utilization of medical treatment services among male Vietnam Veterans. J Nerv Ment Dis 2000; 188(8):496–504.
85. Weisberg RB, Bruce SE, Machan JT, et al. Nonpsychiatric illness among primary care patients with trauma histories and posttraumatic stress disorder. Psychiatr Serv 2002;53(7):848–54.
86. Davidson JR, Weisler RH, Malik ML, et al. Treatment of posttraumatic stress disorder with nefazadone. Int Clin Psychopharmacol 1998;13:111–3.
87. Stein MB, McQuaid JR, Pedrelli P, et al. Posttraumatic stress disorder in the primary care medical setting. Gen Hosp Psychiatry 2000;22:261–9.
88. Magruder KM, Frueh BC, Knapp RG, et al. Prevalence of posttraumatic stress disorder in Veteran Affairs primary care clinics. Gen Hosp Psychiatry 2005;27: 169–79.
89. Burnam MA, Meredith LS, Tanielian T, et al. Mental health care for Iraq and Afghanistan war Veterans. Health Aff (Millwood) 2009;28(3):771–82.
90. Greenberg PE, Sisitsky T, Kessler RC, et al. The economic burden of anxiety disorders in the 1990s. J Clin Psychiatry 1999;60(7):427–35.
91. Kessler RC. Posttraumatic stress disorder: the burden to the individual and to society. J Clin Psychiatry 2000;61(suppl 5):4–12.
92. Lindley SE, Cacciapaglia H, Noronha D, et al. Monitoring mental health treatment acceptance and initial treatment adherence in Veterans: Veterans of Operations Enduring Freedom and Iraqi Freedom versus other Veterans of other eras. Ann N Y Acad Sci 2010;1208:104–13.
93. Harmon AL, Goldstein ES, Shiner B, et al. Preliminary findings for a brief posttraumatic stress intervention in primary mental health care. Psychol Serv 2014;11(3):295–9.
94. Watts BV, Shiner B, Zubkoff L, et al. Implementation of evidence-based psychotherapies for posttraumatic stress disorder in VA specialty clinics. Psychiatr Serv 2014;65(5):648–53.
95. Jakupcak M, Wagner A, Paulson A, et al. Behavioral activation as a primary care-based treatment for PTSD and depression among returning Veterans. J Trauma Stress 2010;23(4):491–5.

96. Wagner A, Zatzick D, Ghesquiere A, et al. Behavioral activation as an early intervention for posttraumatic stress disorder and depression among physically injured trauma survivors. Cogn Behav Pract 2007;14:341–9.

97. Friborg O, Martinussen M, Kaiser S, et al. Comorbidity of personality disorders in anxiety disorders: a meta-analysis of 30 years of research. J Affect Disord 2013;145(2):143–55.

98. Ginzburg K, Ein-Dor T, Solomon Z. Comorbidity of posttraumatic stress disorder, anxiety and depression: a 20-year longitudinal study of war Veterans. J Affect Disord 2010;123(1):249–57.

99. Lockwood E, Forbes D. Posttraumatic stress disorder and comorbidity: untangling the Gordian knot. Psychol Inj Law 2014;7(2):108–21.

100. Mueser KT, Rosenberg SD, Goodman LA, et al. Trauma, PTSD, and the course of severe mental illness: an interactive model. Schizophr Res 2002;53(1–2): 123–43.

101. Brady KT, Dansky BS, Back SE, et al. Exposure therapy in the treatment of PTSD among cocaine-dependent individuals: preliminary findings. J Subst Abuse Treat 2001;21(1):47–54.

102. McGovern MP, Lambert-Harris C, Alterman AI, et al. A randomized controlled trial comparing integrated cognitive behavioral therapy versus individual addiction counseling for co-occurring substance use and posttraumatic stress disorders. J Dual Diagn 2011;7(4):207–27.

103. Hoge CW, McGurk D, Thomas JL, et al. Mild traumatic brain injury in U.S. soldiers returning from Iraq. N Engl J Med 2008;358(5):453–63.

104. Tanev KS, Pentel KZ, Kredlow MA, et al. PTSD and TBI co-morbidity: scope, clinical presentation and treatment options. Brain Inj 2014;28(3):261–70.

105. Chard KM, Schumm JA, McIlvain SM, et al. Exploring the efficacy of a residential treatment program incorporating cognitive processing therapy-cognitive for Veterans with PTSD and traumatic brain injury. J Trauma Stress 2011;24:347–51.

106. Walter KH, Kiefer SL, Chard KM. Relationship between posttraumatic stress disorder and postconcussive symptom improvement after completion of a posttraumatic stress disorder/traumatic brain injury residential treatment program. Rehabil Psychol 2012;57:13–7.

107. Wolf GK, Strom TQ, Kehle SM, et al. A preliminary examination of prolonged exposure therapy with Iraq and Afghanistan Veterans with a diagnosis of posttraumatic stress disorder and mild to moderate traumatic brain injury. J Head Trauma Rehabil 2012;27:26–32.

108. Burke JS, Degeneffe CE, Olney MF. A new disability for rehabilitation counselors: Iraq war Veterans with traumatic brain injury and post-traumatic stress disorder. J Rehabil Med 2009;75:5–14.

109. Panagioti M, Gooding PA, Tarrier N. A meta-analysis of the association between posttraumatic stress disorder and suicidality: the role of comorbid depression. Compr Psychiatry 2012;53(7):915–30.

110. Pompili M, Sher L, Serafini G, et al. Posttraumatic stress disorder and suicide risk among Veterans: a literature review. J Nerv Ment Dis 2013;201(9):802–12.

111. Rice TR, Sher L. Suicidal behavior in war Veterans. Expert Rev Neurother 2012; 12(5):611–24.

112. Jacobs D, Brewer M. APA practice guideline provides recommendations for assessing and treating patients with suicidal behaviors. Psychiatr Ann 2004;34(5): 373–80.

113. Department of Veterans Affairs, Department of Defense. VA/DoD clinical practice guideline for the assessment and management of patients at risk for

suicide. Washington, DC: Department of Veterans Affairs, Department of Defense; 2013.

114. Creech SK, Benzer JK, Liebsack BK, et al. Impact of coping style and PTSD on family functioning after deployment in Operation Desert Shield/Storm returnees. J Trauma Stress 2013;26(4):507–11.

115. Meis LA, Schaaf KW, Erbes CR, et al. Interest in partner-involved services among Veterans seeking mental health care from a VA PTSD clinic. Psychol Trauma 2013;5(4):334–42.

116. Department of Veterans Affairs. Iraq war clinician guide. 2nd edition. Washington, DC: National Center for Post-Traumatic Stress Disorder and Walter Reed Army Medical Center, Department of Veterans Affairs; 2004.

117. Polusny MA, Kumpula MJ, Meis LA, et al. Gender differences in the effects of deployment-related stressors and pre-deployment risk factors on the development of PTSD symptoms in national guard soldiers deployed to Iraq and Afghanistan. J Psychiatr Res 2014;49:1–9.

118. Washington DL, Davis TD, Der-Martirosian C, et al. PTSD risk and mental health care engagement in a multi-war era community sample of women Veterans. J Gen Intern Med 2013;28(7):894–900.

119. Kelly MM, Vogt DS, Scheiderer EM, et al. Effects of military trauma exposure on women Veterans' use and perceptions of Veterans health administration care. J Gen Intern Med 2008;23(6):741–7.

120. Vogt D, Bergeron A, Salgado D, et al. Barriers to Veterans health administration care in a nationally representative sample of women Veterans. J Gen Intern Med 2006;21:S19–25.

121. Federal law, Title 38 U.S. Code 1720D. Veterans Benefits. Counseling and treatment for sexual trauma; 2006.

122. Hoyt T, Rielage JK, Williams LF. Military sexual trauma in men: a review of reported rates. J Trauma Dissociation 2011;12(3):244–60.

123. Turchik JA, Wilson SM. Sexual assault in the U.S. military: a review of the literature and recommendations for the future. Aggression Violent Beh 2010;15(4): 267–77.

124. Kimerling R, Street AE, Pavao J, et al. Military-related sexual trauma among Veterans Health Administration patients returning from Afghanistan and Iraq. Am J Public Health 2010;100(8):1409–12.

125. Surís A, Link-Malcolm J, Chard K, et al. A randomized clinical trial of cognitive processing therapy for Veterans with PTSD related to military sexual trauma. J Trauma Stress 2013;26(1):28–37.

126. Rauch SA, Defever E, Favorite T, et al. Prolonged exposure for PTSD in a Veterans health administration PTSD clinic. J Trauma Stress 2009;22(1):60–4.

127. Noonan M, Mumola C. Veterans in state and federal prison, 2004. Washington, DC: U.S. Department of Justice, Office of Justice Programs, Bureau of Justice Statistics; 2007.

128. Greenberg G, Rosenheck R. Jail incarceration, homelessness, and mental health: a national study. Psychiatr Serv 2008;59:170–7.

129. Weaver CM, Trafton JA, Kimerling R, et al. Prevalence and nature of criminal offending in a national sample of Veterans in VA substance use treatment prior to the operation enduring freedom/operation Iraqi freedom conflicts. Psychol Serv 2013;10(1):54–66.

130. Elbogen EB, Wagner HR, Fuller SR, et al. Correlates of anger and hostility in Iraq and Afghanistan war veterans. Am J Psychiatry 2010;167(9):1051–8.

Intimate Partner Violence

The Role of Nurses in Protection of Patients

Lisa N. Hewitt, RN, MSN, APRN-BC, ACNP

KEYWORDS

- Intimate partner violence • Domestic violence • Nursing • Social action
- Violence against women

KEY POINTS

- If healthcare is going to stop the cycle of violence and prevent the killing of women, it is imperative that all healthcare systems develop protocols for the training of professionals to routinely screen and intervene for patients who are associated with a violent partner; these protocols should be followed and included in the departmental and hospital quality improvement programs.
- It is the responsibility of healthcare professionals to identify, intervene, and advocate for intimate partner violence (IPV) victims when they present to an emergency department or healthcare setting.
- Using a 20 s screening tool (PVS) and asking questions in a nonjudgemental manner can quickly and easily be the difference between life and death for many women.

INTRODUCTION

Federal Bureau of Investigation statistics have shown that a woman is beaten every 18 seconds[1] and 4 out of every 10 women in the United States are likely to have experienced some form of violence during their lifetime.[2] Although women experience fewer violent crimes overall than men, they are five to eight times more likely than men to be victimized or killed by an intimate partner.[3] Not only do women experience intimate partner violence (IPV) more often than men, they are many times repeatedly victimized by the same partner.[4]

IPV is defined as any behavior within an intimate relationship that causes physical, psychological, or sexual harm to those in the relationship. These behaviors include, but are not limited to physical violence, sexual violence, psychological abuse, and controlling behaviors.[5] IPV not only causes immediate injury to women, but can also have long-term

Disclosures: No disclosure and no trademarks.
Department of Trauma and Disaster Management, Parkland Hospital, 5201 Harry Hines Boulevard, Dallas, TX 75235, USA
E-mail address: Lisa.Hewitt@phhs.org

Crit Care Nurs Clin N Am 27 (2015) 271–275
http://dx.doi.org/10.1016/j.cnc.2015.02.004
0899-5885/15/$ – see front matter © 2015 Elsevier Inc. All rights reserved.

ccnursing.theclinics.com

sequela for women including depression, suicide, substance abuse, gastrointestinal disorders, and chronic pain syndromes.[6] Health care settings and specifically nurses are primary avenues for victim identification and intervention for female survivors of IPV.[7]

HISTORICAL REVIEW

IPV has been part of the common vernacular for centuries; during the Reformation a common saying was "Women, like walnut trees, should be beaten every day."[8] In 1824 in Mississippi laws were passed legalizing wife-beating. It was legal in every state in the United States for men to rape their wives until the 1970s. There were laws in the United States preserving the legality of marital rape until the early 1990s.[8] In 1985, the Surgeon General identified IPV as a public health problem of epidemic proportions with IPV resulting in 30% of homicides.[7] In 1992, the Joint Commission on Accreditation of Healthcare Organizations established guidelines that required accredited hospitals to implement policies and procedures in their emergency department and ambulatory care settings for identifying, treating, and referring victims of abuse,[9] but detection is still not to the degree necessary.[10] Despite these advances in laws "the response of the healthcare community to domestic violence had been slow and inconsistent."[11]

INCIDENCE

The actual incidence of IPV is unknown, because of underreporting of the violence by the victim, and of underinvestigation by law enforcement and health care workers. In the United States, an estimated of 36 million women have experienced violence as a child or an adult.[2] Almost 30% of women worldwide have been in a relationship where they have experienced physical or sexual violence by their intimate partner.[12] Persons may be victims of IPV and no one may know it, other than the victim and abuser. The National Violence Against Women Survey[12] estimates that

- 5.3 million women 18 years old and older are victims of IPV every year
- Two million injuries occur at the hands of abusers
- Eight million days of lost work because of IPV
- $4.1 billion annually is paid for direct medical care and mental health services because of IPV

INTIMATE PARTNER VIOLENCE AND MORTALITY

It is not uncommon for IPV to lead to death. Intimate partner homicide is the single largest category of female homicide with women most often being killed by a husband, lover, ex-husband, or ex-lover.[13] Homicide is also the leading cause of pregnancy-associated death.[14] Most women that are killed by IPV have been abused before being murdered by their partner.[13] The odds of a female victim dying from firearm violence are 10 times higher when shot by an intimate partner than when shot by a stranger.[15]

LONG-TERM EFFECTS

Immediate physical injury is the stereotypical presentation associated with IPV, but women face more than physical scars. Victims of IPV are at an increased risk for chronic health problems that arise from prolonged stress.[5] Abused women are two times more likely than nonabused women to report poor health, both physical and mental, even if the violence occurred many years in the past. The incidence of drug and alcohol abuse, eating and sleeping disorders, physical inactivity, poor self-esteem, posttraumatic stress disorder, smoking, self-harm, and unsafe sexual behavior are also increased.[5] Thoughts of suicide and attempted suicide are significantly higher among women who have experienced this violence.[5] Women who experience intimate sexual violence are four to five times more likely to suffer from anxiety and depression than women who have not experienced violence.[2]

LEAVING THE ABUSER

Many health care professionals have preconceived ideas as to why women do not leave their abusers, but often it is more complicated. Women are not passive victims in their abuse; many times they adopt strategies to maximize their safety and the safety of their children. A woman's response to abuse is often related to the options available to her.[5] There are multiple reasons why women stay in a violent relationship. Often it is fear of retaliation from the abuser. She may not have any other economic means for support of herself and/or her children. Other reasons for staying with the abuser may be concern for her children; lack of support from family and friends; stigma or fear of losing custody of children associated with divorce; and love, with the hope that her partner will change.[5] When women do leave, it is often after multiple attempts to leave and many years of violence.[5]

STOPPING THE VIOLENCE

The first step to stopping IPV is diagnosing the problem. Often it is difficult to diagnosis IPV by injuries alone. Studies have shown victims of IPV most commonly have head and neck injuries, with the head being the most common site for lethal gunshot wounds from IPV,[16] followed by musculoskeletal injuries.[17] However, 58.3% of total IPV patients presenting to emergency departments within 1 year of their death presented with non–injury-related problems.[16] In one study the presenting complaint for victims of IPV was falls, with that being the highest rate of injury for women aged 15 to 44.[18] Victims of IPV are not always forthcoming about their injuries, but they are not offended when asked in a nonjudgmental or nondemeaning manner.[10] It is important to accurately document what has happened, which includes the physical examination and written documentation. It is critical to be as specific as possible when documenting the physical examination.

The Partner Violence Screen (PVS) (**Box 1**) is a validated three question-screening tool that is easy to use and quick to score. An answer of "yes" to any of the three PVS screening questions is considered a positive screen. The PVS detects heterosexual and homosexual partner abuse.[19]

In the trauma patient population it has been shown that attaching the PVS to the Screening, Brief, Intervention, and Referral for Treatment (SBIRT) was significantly better at detecting IPV than a nurse-performed screen. SBIRT is drug and alcohol screening mandated by the American College of Surgeons for trauma center verification. Combining the screening eased the busy role of nursing by linking the PVS to SBIRT, which is protocol driven and a quality improvement indicator for the trauma program.[20]

Box 1
Partner violence screen

1. Have you been kicked, hit, punched, or otherwise hurt by someone in the past year? If so, by whom?

2. Do you feel safe in your current relationship?

3. Is there a partner from a previous relationship who is making you feel unsafe now?

It is important to maximize the safety of the victim by doing an interview in private, without the partner or family present. Screening for IPV in the presence of other family members is not only futile, but it may put the victim at risk of injury if the partner is informed and intervenes to silence the victim.[10]

More women who were killed by intimate partners sought help in a health care setting than any other helping agencies. Thus, health care professionals have the unique position to identify victims of IPV and potentially prevent tragedy.[13] Health care settings and nurses are primary avenues for identification and intervention for female survivors of IPV. Universal screening is advocated as an approach to increase identification partly because no demographic profile, pattern of injuries, or clinical illness can reliably identified women affected by IPV.[7]

Strategically placed posters, brochures, skills training for providers, and routine questions about IPV on health questionnaires have been shown to increase awareness in providers and increase detection of IPV. Specifically, wall posters portray valuable information without signaling out a specific woman in the presence of the abuser. The restroom is one location an abuser is likely not allowed to go with the victim, making this an ideal location for brochures and posters.[21]

Education programs are needed for all health care professionals, not just in obstetrics and gynecology offices, and in the emergency departments. Victims interact with all facets of the health care system and all health care workers should be aware of the need to screen for IPV. If health care workers can screen for IPV and provide interventions for the victims, there should be a subsequent decline in the death rates of the abused.

SUMMARY

Many people entering into the health care field do so to help people. Using a quick screening tool, brochures, and/or posters is a fast and easy way to not only help people, but more importantly to save someone's life. If women's safety is to be promoted, the cycle of abuse interrupted, and the killing of women prevented, it is imperative that all health care agencies develop protocols for the training of professionals to routinely screen and intervene for patients who are associated with a violent partner.[13] These protocols should be followed and included in the departmental and hospital quality improvement programs.

Many victims of IPV present to the emergency department at least once and sometimes multiple times within a year before their murder,[16] and it is the responsibility of health care professionals to identify, intervene, and advocate for these patients. Using a 20-second screening tool (PVS) and asking questions in a nonjudgmental manner can quickly and easily be the difference between life and death for many women. The victim may not identify her attacker initially, but if the health care provider continues to show her that the health care environment is a safe place, perhaps she will be able to share her painful secret. Health care professionals must not let their own biases and judgments affect the care they provide. It is their job to help and save the victims of IPV.

REFERENCES

1. Moore D. Battered women. 1st edition. Oakbrook Terrace (IL): Sage Publications; 1979.
2. Plichta SB, Falik M. Prevalence of violence and its implications for women's health. Womens Health Issues 2001;11:244–58.
3. Greenfeld LA, Rand MR, Craven D, et al. Violence by intimates: analysis of data on crimes by current or former spouses, boyfriends, and girlfriends. Bureau of

Justice Statistics Factbook. 1998. NCJ-167237. Available at: http://bjs.gov/content/pub/pdf/vi.pdf.

4. Tjaden P, Thoennes N. Extent, nature, and consequences of IPV: findings from the national violence against women survey [Electronic version]. Washington, DC: U.S. Department of Justice, Office of Justice Programs, National Institute of Justice and the Center for Disease Control; 2000. Available at: https://www.ncjrs.gov/pdffiles1/nij/181867.pdf. Accessed November 29, 2014.

5. World Health Organization. Understanding and addressing violence against women: intimate partner violence [Fact Sheet]. 2012. Available at: http://apps.who.int/iris/bitstream/10665/77432/1/WHO_RHR_12.36_eng.pdf?ua=1. Accessed November 1, 2014.

6. Heise L, Garcia-Moreno C. World report on violence and health: violence by intimate partners. Geneva (Switzerland): World Health Organization; 2002.

7. Walton-Moss B, Campbell JC. Intimate partner violence: implications for nursing. Online J Issues Nurs 2002;7:6. Available at: http://www.nursingworld.org/MainMenurCategories/ANAMarketplace/ANAPPeriodicals/OJIN/TableofContents/Volume72002/No1Jan2002/IntimatePartnerViolence.html.

8. Kelly U. Theories of IPV: from blaming the victim to acting against injustice: intersectionality as an analytic framework. ANS Adv Nurs Sci 2011;34:E29–51.

9. Johnson BJ. Intimate partner violence screening and treatment: the importance of caring behaviors. J Forensic Nurs 2006;2:184–8.

10. Griffin MP, Koss MP. Clinical screening and intervention in cases of partner violence. Online J Issues Nurs 2002;7:3. Available at: http://www.nursingworld.org/MainMenurCategories/ANAMarketplace/ANAPPeriodicals/OJIN/TableofContents/Volume72002/No1Jan2002/ClinicalScreeningandPartnerViolence.html.

11. Flitcraft A. Physicians and domestic violence: challenges for prevention. Health Aff (Millwood) 1993;12:155–61.

12. World Health Organization, Department of Reproductive Health and Research (2013). Global and regional estimates of violence against women: prevalence and health effects of intimate partner violence and non-partner sexual violence (WHO Reference Number 978 92 4 156462 5). Available at: http://apps.who.int/iris/bitstream/10665/85239/1/9789241564625_eng.pdf. Accessed November 1, 2014.

13. Sharps PW, Koziol-McLain J, Campbell J, et al. Health care providers' missed opportunities for preventing femicide. Prev Med 2001;33:373–80.

14. Horon IL, Cheng D. Enhanced surveillance for pregnancy-associated mortality—Maryland, 1993-1998. JAMA 2001;285:1455–9.

15. Finlay-Morreale HE, Tsuei BJ, Fisher BS, et al. Close is dead: determinants of firearm injury lethality in women. J Trauma 2009;66:1207–11.

16. Wadman MC, Muelleman RL. Domestic violence homicides: ED use before victimization. Am J Emerg Med 1999;17:689–91.

17. Bhandari M, Dosanjh S, Tornette P, et al. Musculoskeletal manifestations of physical abuse after intimate partner violence. J Trauma 2006;61:1473–9.

18. Grisso JA, Wishner AR, Schwartz DF, et al. A population-based study of injuries in inner-city women. Am J Epidemiol 1991;134:59–86.

19. Feldhaus K, Koziol-McLain J, Amsbury H, et al. Accuracy of 3 brief screening questions for detecting partner violence in the emergency department. JAMA 1997;277:1357–61.

20. Hewitt LN, Bhavsar P, Phelan HA. The secrets women keep: intimate partner violence screening in the female trauma patient. J Trauma 2011;70(2):320–3.

21. Thompson RS, Rivara PF, Thompson DC, et al. Identification and management of domestic violence: a randomized trial. Am J Prev Med 2000;19(4):253–63.

Blast Injury

Impact on Brain and Internal Organs

Richard N. Lesperance, MD[a],*, Timothy C. Nunez, MD, FACS[a,b]

KEYWORDS

- Blast injury • Polytrauma • Terrorism • Traumatic brain injury

KEY POINTS

- Injuries caused by blast effects may be incurred by both soldiers during wartime and civilians involved in terrorist incidents or industrial accidents.
- The injuries caused by blast are usually divided into primary (blast overpressure), secondary (fragmentation), tertiary (blunt trauma), and quaternary (burns, toxic exposures) effects.
- The most commonly injured systems are the lungs, brain, and extremities.
- Brain damage may be subtle but a source of long-term impairment.

INTRODUCTION

The use of explosives to kill and injure soldiers by blast effects probably goes back a thousand years, to the introduction of gunpowder to warfare. During the recent military conflicts in Iraq and Afghanistan, a higher proportion of casualties were caused by blast injuries compared with previous conflicts, because of the widespread adoption of improvised explosive devices (IEDs) by enemy forces.[1,2] Coupled with a decreased case fatality rate,[3] this means that a larger number of survivors of blast injuries have been treated in military and Veteran's Administration medical systems, which has brought increasing appreciation of the long-term effects of blast injury on the brain, even in less severely injured casualties.

Outside wartime, injuries caused by blast remain a threat to civilians as well. IEDs are a favorite weapon of terrorists, from nineteenth century bomb-throwing anarchists to the perpetrators of the recent Boston Marathon bombings. Major terrorist incidents

Disclosures: The authors have nothing to disclose.
[a] Division of Trauma and Surgical Critical Care, Vanderbilt University Medical Center, 1211 21st Avenue South, 404 Medical Arts Building, Nashville, TN 37212-1750, USA; [b] Department of Surgery, Tennessee Valley VA Medical Center, 1310 24th Avenue South, Nashville, TN 37212-1750, USA
* Corresponding author. Department of Surgery, Tennessee Valley VA Medical Center, Nashville, TN 37212-1750.
E-mail address: richard.n.lesperance@vanderbilt.edu

Crit Care Nurs Clin N Am 27 (2015) 277–287
http://dx.doi.org/10.1016/j.cnc.2015.02.007
0899-5885/15/$ – see front matter Published by Elsevier Inc.

of the twentieth and twenty-first centuries have relied on IEDs to kill and terrorize, be it a hijacked airplane or a gunpowder-laden pressure-cooker. In addition, industrial accidents such as the West Texas fertilizer plant explosion in 2013 can injure a large number of people by blast effects, with a similar injury pattern to military or terrorist casualties.

CLASSIFICATION OF BLAST EFFECTS

The effects of an explosive blast are generally grouped into 4 categories (**Table 1**) that are considered separately here.

Primary Blast Effects

Primary blast effects are those caused by the overpressure wave of the explosion. The blast wave propagates in 3 dimensions, and decreases in force as it travels farther from the source. However, when encountering a structure or when confined inside a building, the blast wave can be subject to complex and unpredictable changes in its destructive force,[4] and proximity to the blast does not always correlate with injury severity.[5] The orientation of the casualty to the blast (ie, facing toward or sideways) can also influence the injuries received.[4] Reviews of military casualties from Iraq and Afghanistan reveal more severe primary blast injuries among personnel inside vehicles,[6] suggesting that armored vehicles may protect against secondary fragmentation damage but still transmit a significant overpressure wave.

Organs frequently injured by primary blast injury (PBI) include the lungs, tympanic membranes (TMs), intestines, and brain. Isolated PBI may not leave any external signs of injury in a casualty, requiring a high index of suspicion to identify these injuries. PBI causes injury primarily in air-filled organs and at air-fluid interfaces. As the blast wave propagates through the casualty, barotrauma or change in pressure at these interfaces causes injury. Solid organs are also susceptible to barotrauma but in general require the casualty to be very close to the center of the blast. Cardiac dysfunction can occur either because of a direct myocardial depressant effect or arrhythmias.[7–9] In addition, PBI to vascular endothelium may cause diffuse plasma leakage and resultant hemoconcentration and hypovolemic shock, even in the absence of other injuries causing blood loss.[10]

Classically, a ruptured TM was seen as a marker for blast severity, and a normal otoscopic examination was thought to identify a patient at low risk for PBI. This concept has not been supported by data from recent incidents. In a review of injuries from the 2004 Madrid train bombings, only approximately 50% of the casualties had ruptured TMs (although this study did not differentiate between primary and secondary blast injuries).[11] In another study, investigators studied a series of military blast casualties in Iraq, and found that only 16% had perforated TMs. When they analyzed injuries that could only be caused by primary blast effects (eg, simple pneumothorax, pulmonary contusion), they still only had 50% with ruptured TMs.[12] Given this, we do not think that a normal otoscopic examination can exclude a significant PBI.

Table 1 Types of blast injuries	
Primary	Injuries caused directly by blast overpressure wave
Secondary	Fragmentation injuries
Tertiary	Blunt trauma caused by displacement of the casualty, or structural collapse
Quaternary	Burns, toxic inhalation, chemical exposure, or radiation exposure

Secondary Blast Effects

Secondary blast effects are those caused by fragments propelled by the initial explosion. Military munitions such as hand grenades and artillery shells are frequently engineered to use metal fragments to increase their lethality. The design of an IED can deliberately incorporate nails, bolts, or other metal fragments for the same reason (such as those used for the Boston Marathon bombing). In addition, material near the blast epicenter can form incidental secondary projectiles. The authors have frequently identified gravel, glass, and metal fragments of vehicles causing secondary fragment injuries in combat casualties they have treated. Secondary blast injury to the extremities is a common injury pattern in recent military as well as civilian casualties, resulting in severe bone and soft tissue wounds.[13,14]

Disturbingly, biological material can form secondary projectiles that cause injury in survivors, both from the perpetrators of human-borne IEDs (suicide bombers) and also from other casualties located closer to the blast epicenter.[15,16] This material can transmit infectious diseases, and may be a source of psychological distress to the casualty because of the nature of its origin.

Tertiary Blast Effects

The blast wave created by the explosion can propel casualties away from the blast site, causing blunt force trauma when the casualties strike the ground or other object in their path. In addition, crush injuries from building collapse are considered tertiary blast trauma as well. The contribution of these injuries can vary significantly between different incidents. For example, in the Oklahoma City bombing, most survivors had crush injuries, whereas after the September 11 attacks on the World Trade Center, the collapse of the towers ensured that very few casualties sustaining crush injuries survived.[17,18]

Quaternary Blast Effects

This category of effects describes the impact of burns, toxic inhalants, and other exposures. Burns accompanying significant trauma from secondary or tertiary effects magnify the management problems involved.[19] Dust and other inhaled toxins generated by explosives or structural collapse can be a significant source of morbidity in survivors. For example, although only 1% of survivors from the collapse of the World Trade Center had crush injuries, up to 50% of them were treated for inhalation injuries.[17] In addition, there are significant concerns remaining about the effects of the inhaled particulates on the long-term health of both survivors and rescuers. Industrial accidents present the possibility of toxic chemicals used in chemical processes or as products of combustion from the explosion or subsequent fires.

A particularly morbid aspect of quaternary blast effects is the concept of the so-called dirty bomb, in which low-grade radiologic material is placed in the IED to be dispersed by the explosion. The radioactive material may be enough to cause radiation sickness in exposed people, complicate cleanup efforts, or just act as a psychological weapon to increase anxiety among the public.[20,21] Some authorities prefer to include deliberate additives to IEDs in a separate category of quinary blast effects.[22]

PRESENTATION AND INITIAL TRIAGE

Whether it is a terrorist incident or an industrial accident, there typically is scant notice before the arrival of the initial casualties. Less severely injured casualties who are able to seek medical care under their own power are likely to arrive first, before more seriously injured patients are assessed, triaged, and transported by the emergency medical system (EMS). This process has been termed an upside-down triage[23] but, depending on local circumstances, it may not always be seen. Because of a robust EMS response, seriously injured casualties from the Boston Marathon bombings were transported to Boston trauma centers within 15 minutes of the attack.[24] Typically, about one-half of the total casualties present in the first hour after the incident, and this rule can be used to estimate the total number of injured,[23] but structure collapse and the need for extrication can delay the arrival of seriously injured patients.[18] Communication with EMS at the scene can provide valuable information about possible delayed arrival of seriously injured patients, as well as complicating details like structure collapse. In addition, EMS and local fire department personnel can provide valuable information as to the risk of quaternary inhalational injury during industrial accidents by identifying the chemical risk involved.

RESUSCITATION

Blast casualties, by their nature, tend to be patients with multisystem trauma who should be managed in accordance with the principles of Advanced Trauma Life Support (ATLS). Severe extremity wounds from secondary fragments or crush injuries can be dramatic but should not distract from managing the casualty's airway, oxygenation, and circulatory status.

Some blast casualties benefit from damage control resuscitation (DCR). Of all patients who arrive at civilian trauma centers only about 3% require a massive transfusion or DCR.[25] Military casualties, who are involved in exponentially more blast injuries, have a higher rate of need for DCR.[26] The term damage control has now become standard phraseology describing a variety of surgical tactics and techniques applicable across a wide range of surgical disciplines, including orthopedic surgery, neurosurgery, emergency general surgery, vascular surgery ophthalmic surgery, urologic surgery, and burn surgery.[27] The term damage control has also now been extended to both the prehospital and early resuscitation phase and is sometimes termed damage control zero (DC 0).[28–30] DC 0 is prehospital DCR. DC 0 is applied early, typically before hospital arrival, with the goal of keeping the patient out of trouble. DCR directly addresses the lethal triad because it is often fatal for patients to become cold, coagulopathic, and acidotic.[31] Prehospital providers need to be proficient in identifying casualties who require this DCR approach. It may be difficult for providers to rapidly identify this group of patients. Although there are no uniformly accepted criteria to identify the patients who will benefit from DCR, several groups have developed scoring systems (using a variety of anatomic, physiologic, and laboratory variables) to correctly identify the patients who are likely to require a massive transfusion.[32–35] Although each of these scoring systems is quite accurate, there are 2 scoring systems that are most applicable to EMS. They can use these scores to assist their clinical acumen in selecting out this critical group of patients.[32,35] The tenets of DCR are limited crystalloid resuscitation, permissive hypotension, hemostatic resuscitation, and proper patient selection.[26,28,32,35–37]

REVIEW OF SPECIFIC INJURIES
Lungs

Because of the nature of the lung, involving countless air/fluid interfaces, it is particularly sensitive to the overpressure injury of PBI. Diffuse alveolar and parenchymal hemorrhage is the hallmark disorder on autopsy.[38] Unlike other categories of blast injury, PBI to the lung does not present with any obvious external findings, so medical personnel must be alert to its possibility in the setting of pulmonary decline in a blast casualty. The most common presentation is worsening hypoxia with the characteristic butterfly appearance of central bilateral infiltrates on plain radiographs (**Fig. 1**) or computed tomography.[39]

Treatment is supportive: many patients require mechanical ventilation, but, for casualties who are oxygenating adequately 2 hours after injury, further deterioration is rare.[39] Conventional ventilation with a low-tidal-volume strategy seems to work well for these patients, but there are no randomized trials comparing different strategies. High-frequency oscillatory ventilation and extracorporeal membrane oxygenation may work as rescue therapies in refractory patients.[39–41] Patients with PBI to the lung may also present with a simple pneumothorax, pneumomediastinum, or (in rare cases) air embolism that may cause neurologic symptoms.[39]

Extremity Wounds

These can be the most dramatic injuries, and pose management challenges because of their complex nature, but are rarely a cause of early death in blast injury casualties. Tissue damage to the extremities can be caused by all 4 blast effects but secondary (fragmentation) and tertiary (crush and blunt trauma) mechanisms predominate. Casualties whose extremity injuries are caused by primary blast effects have an extremely high mortality from associated injuries because of the force involved.[14]

The combinations of blast damage, fragmentation, crush, and burns complicate wound management (**Fig. 2**). In the military setting, they are frequently accompanied by genitourinary or pelvic injuries,[42] areas not well protected by modern battle armor. Among civilian casualties of similar blasts, injury to the unprotected torso can also be expected.

During initial management of casualties, tourniquets should be used liberally for concerns about extremity hemorrhage. Even if a limb does not have current, active arterial hemorrhage, resuscitation of the casualty can overcome arterial vasospasm and cause recurrent hemorrhage. EMS personnel should carry tourniquets and have a low threshold for their use in multiply injured patients with trauma.[43] If not placed in the field, they should be placed in the emergency department for casualties with significant extremity wounds at risk for arterial hemorrhage; in the setting of a mass-casualty scenario, recurrent hemorrhage might not be noticed promptly. Historical concerns about the safety of tourniquet use have mainly been disproved. Tourniquets have been used and studied extensively during the recent conflicts in Iraq and

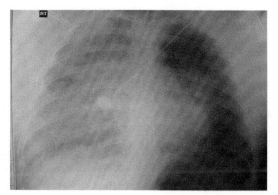

Fig. 1. Characteristic butterfly appearance of central bilateral infiltrates on plain radiograph.

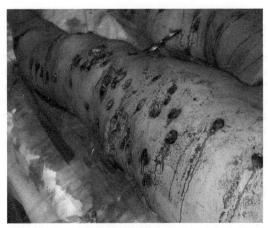

Fig. 2. Combination of blast damage, fragmentation, crush injury, and burns.

Afghanistan,[44,45] and they have been found to be generally safe and very effective at saving lives. It is now widely accepted to use tourniquets in the prehospital arena. Tourniquet use is now taught in both the civilian and military versions of Pre-Hospital Trauma Life Support. As mentioned previously, DCR should be practiced until major extremity vascular injury is either excluded or surgically controlled.

Complex extremity wounds should undergo early evaluation and debridement as soon as the casualty is appropriately resuscitated. All nonviable tissue needs to be debrided from the wounds to decrease risk of wound infection and bioburden from dead tissue.[46] Definitive fracture fixation and wound closure/soft tissue coverage does not need to be done emergently, and delays to definitive closure of up to 12 days are not associated with an increase in infectious complications.[47]

All casualties with any penetrating injury from blast effects should have their tetanus status checked and updated if necessary. Prophylactic antibiotics are absolutely indicated in the setting of open fractures and should be directed against common skin flora.[48] Embedded biological fragments should be surgically removed and the casualty should receive immunization for hepatitis B and have serum samples archived for future hepatitis C and human immunodeficiency virus testing.[15]

Trauma Brain Injury

Blast injury to the brain ranges from immediately lethal injuries to mild impairment that may initially go unnoticed. Secondary fragmentation may cause penetrating injury to any portion of the brain, and tertiary blast effects can cause closed head injuries similar to those seen in patients with conventional blunt trauma.[49,50] In addition, primary blast effects can have a range of consequences to the brain that have only recently become appreciated. Focal neurologic deficits can be caused by air embolisms as sequelae of lung injury.[50] The primary blast wave can cause sinus fractures, as well as intracranial cavitation and shear injuries that can cause neuronal damage, and disrupt the capillary blood-brain barrier.[51] The resulting diffuse axonal injury (DAI) may be functionally different from injuries resulting from focal trauma.[52]

There has been increasing awareness of the presence and importance of mild TBI (mTBI) in the last few years because of the concussive effects of PBI to the brain. This injury has been termed the signature wound of the wars in Iraq and Afghanistan, and despite the subtle symptoms can pose a significant quality-of-life burden.[53] Casualties may experience retrograde amnesia, headaches, confusion, altered executive function/decision making, mood disturbances, and sleep alterations.[54] Although conventional brain imaging involving computed tomography and MRI is often negative in these patients, specialized scanning technologies have detected signs of DAI in even minimally symptomatic patients with mTBI.[55] In addition, there seems to be significant overlap in symptoms between patients with mTBI and casualties (both military and civilian) with posttraumatic stress disorder, and epidemiologic reviews suggest a causative relationship.[56] Several questionnaire-based screening tools have been developed to identify mTBI.[53,57,58] Identification of casualties with even mTBI is important because of the benefits of cognitive rehabilitation and the need to provide support for what may be lifelong, if subtle, neurocognitive problems.[59,60]

Rehabilitation and Outcomes

Individuals with significant injuries related to blast trauma should be evaluated for rehabilitation after their acute injuries are stabilized.[61] Even aside from obvious needs like prostheses for amputated limbs, both military and civilian casualties of blast trauma may have lifelong disability because of the complex nature of their injuries.[60]

For blast injuries to the extremities, the greater wound complexity and tissue damage suggest a worse prognosis compared with other mechanisms. However, a recent study comparing upper extremity blast injuries with gunshot wounds in casualties of terrorism revealed similar functional outcomes and ultimate quality of life, despite more complex wounds.[62]

Brain injury has an obvious effect on ultimate functional status and rehabilitative potential. Even mTBI has been associated with lower functional quality of life and return to work after rehabilitation.[63–66] Casualties who have additional injuries as a result of blast trauma have more rehabilitation needs than those with isolated head injuries.[67]

Casualties of multiple injuries caused by blast effects may benefit from comprehensive, longitudinal case management to assist in accessing reconstructive and rehabilitative services, as well as identifying more subtle injuries (eg, mTBI) not readily apparent at the initial wounding.[68,69] In addition, for those injured on military service or during certain large-scale terrorist incidents, financial support may be available in different forms to defray living expenses and for caregiver support.

SUMMARY

Blast injury is a threat both to soldiers during wartime and civilians attacked during terrorist incidents or injured during industrial accidents. PBI may cause significant trauma to air-filled (lung) and solid organs (brain), sometimes without significant evidence of external trauma but still with lethal or severe long-term effects. Extremity injuries predominate in military casualties from fragmentation because of the success of modern body armor. Secondary fragmentation also causes significant extremity injuries in civilians but the torso and head are typically exposed. Tertiary blast injury results in significant blunt/crush injuries. Quaternary blast injury can be broad, with burns, radiation, and chemical warfare resulting in significant injuries as well, potentially causing panic among civilian populations. Each category of blast injury can result in severe visible and invisible wounds. TBI is a signature example of the latter. These wounds require long-term care and most patients benefit from long-term rehabilitation and support.

REFERENCES

1. Belmont PJ Jr, McCriskin BJ, Sieg RN, et al. Combat wounds in Iraq and Afghanistan from 2005 to 2009. J Trauma Acute Care Surg 2012;73(1):3–12.

2. Eskridge SL, Macera CA, Galarneau MR, et al. Injuries from combat explosions in Iraq: injury type, location, and severity. Injury 2012;43(10):1678–82.

3. Kelly JF, Ritenour AE, McLaughlin DF, et al. Injury severity and causes of death from Operation Iraqi Freedom and Operation Enduring Freedom: 2003-2004 versus 2006. J Trauma 2008;64(2 Suppl):S21–6 [discussion: S26–7].

4. Stuhmiller J, Phillips YY, Richmond DR. The physics and mechanisms of primary blast injury. In: Zajtchuk R, Bellamy RF, Quick CM, editors. Conventional warfare: ballistic, blast and burn injuries. Washington, DC: Office of the Surgeon General; 1992. p. 241–70.

5. Cooper GJ, Maynard RL, Cross NL, et al. Casualties from terrorist bombings. J Trauma 1983;23(11):955–67.

6. Singleton JA, Gibb IE, Bull AM, et al. Primary blast lung injury prevalence and fatal injuries from explosions: insights from postmortem computed tomographic analysis of 121 improvised explosive device fatalities. J Trauma Acute Care Surg 2013;75(2 Suppl 2):S269–74.

7. Irwin RJ, Lerner MR, Bealer JF, et al. Cardiopulmonary physiology of primary blast injury. J Trauma 1997;43(4):650–5.

8. Guy RJ, Watkins PE, Edmondstone WM. Electrocardiographic changes following primary blast injury to the thorax. J R Nav Med Serv 2000;86(3):125–33.

9. Ozer O, Sari I, Davutoglu V, et al. Pericardial tamponade consequent to a dynamite explosion: blast overpressure injury without penetrating trauma. Tex Heart Inst J 2009;36(3):259–60.

10. Zhang B, Wang A, Hu W, et al. Hemoconcentration caused by microvascular dysfunction after blast injuries to the chest and abdomen of rabbits. J Trauma 2011;71(3):694–701.

11. Turegano-Fuentes F, Caba-Doussoux P, Jover-Navalon JM, et al. Injury patterns from major urban terrorist bombings in trains: the Madrid experience. World J Surg 2008;32(6):1168–75.

12. Harrison CD, Bebarta VS, Grant GA. Tympanic membrane perforation after combat blast exposure in Iraq: a poor biomarker of primary blast injury. J Trauma 2009;67(1):210–1.

13. Covey DC, Born CT. Blast injuries: mechanics and wounding patterns. J Surg Orthop Adv 2010;19(1):8–12.

14. Weil YA, Mosheiff R, Liebergall M. Blast and penetrating fragment injuries to the extremities. J Am Acad Orthop Surg 2006;14(10 Spec No):S136–9.

15. Patel HD, Dryden S, Gupta A, et al. Human body projectiles implantation in victims of suicide bombings and implications for health and emergency care providers: the 7/7 experience. Ann R Coll Surg Engl 2012;94(5):313–7.

16. Eshkol Z, Katz K. Injuries from biologic material of suicide bombers. Injury 2005; 36(2):271–4.

17. CDC. MMWR Weekly. [webpage]. 2002; 1–5. Available at: www.cdc.gov/mmwr/preview/mmwrhtml/mm5101a1.htm. Accessed 16 October, 2014.

18. Mallonee S, Shariat S, Stennies G, et al. Physical injuries and fatalities resulting from the Oklahoma City bombing. JAMA 1996;276(5):382–7.

19. Sheridan RL, Greenhalgh D. Special problems in burns. Surg Clin North Am 2014;94(4):781–91.

20. Commission USNR. Fact sheet on dirty bombs. 2014. Available at: http://www.nrc.gov/reading-rm/doc-collections/fact-sheets/fs-dirty-bombs.html. Accessed 4 November, 2014.

21. Hall RC, Chapman MJ. Medical and psychiatric casualties caused by conventional and radiological (dirty) bombs. Gen Hosp Psychiatry 2006;28(3):242–8.

22. Champion HR, Holcomb JB, Young LA. Injuries from explosions: physics, biophysics, pathology, and required research focus. J Trauma 2009;66(5): 1468–77 [discussion: 1477].

23. CDC. Explosions and blast injuries, a primer for clinicians. 2014. Available at: http://emergency.cdc.gov/masscasualties/explosions.asp. Accessed 16 October, 2014.

24. Boston Trauma Center Chiefs' Collaborative. Boston marathon bombings: an after-action review. J Trauma Acute Care Surg 2014;77(3):501–3.

25. Como JJ, Dutton RP, Scalea TM, et al. Blood transfusion rates in the care of acute trauma. Transfusion 2004;44(6):809–13.

26. Holcomb JB, Jenkins D, Rhee P, et al. Damage control resuscitation: directly addressing the early coagulopathy of trauma. J Trauma 2007;62(2):307–10.

27. Chovanes J, Cannon JW, Nunez TC. The evolution of damage control surgery. Surg Clin North Am 2012;92(4):859–75 vii-viii.

28. Beekley AC. Damage control resuscitation: a sensible approach to the exsanguinating surgical patient. Crit Care Med 2008;36(7):S267–74.

29. Johnson JW, Gracias VH, Schwab CW, et al. Evolution in damage control for exsanguinating penetrating abdominal injury. J Trauma 2001;51(2):261–9 [discussion: 269–71].

30. Le Noel A, Merat S, Ausset S, et al. The damage control resuscitation concept. Ann Fr Anesth Reanim 2011;30(9):665–78 [in French].

31. Moore EE. Thomas G. Orr Memorial Lecture. Staged laparotomy for the hypothermia, acidosis, and coagulopathy syndrome. Am J Surg 1996;172(5): 405–10.

32. Nunez TC, Voskresensky IV, Dossett LA, et al. Early prediction of massive transfusion in trauma: simple as ABC (assessment of blood consumption)? J Trauma 2009;66(2):346–52.

33. McLaughlin DF, Niles SE, Salinas J, et al. A predictive model for massive transfusion in combat casualty patients. J Trauma 2008;64(2 Suppl):S57–63 [discussion: S63].

34. Yucel N, Lefering R, Maegele M, et al. Trauma Associated Severe Hemorrhage (TASH)-Score: probability of mass transfusion as surrogate for life threatening hemorrhage after multiple trauma. J Trauma 2006;60(6):1228–36 [discussion: 1236–7].

35. Vandromme MJ, Griffin RL, Kerby JD, et al. Identifying risk for massive transfusion in the relatively normotensive patient: utility of the prehospital shock index. J Trauma 2011;70(2):384–8 [discussion: 388–90].

36. Bickell WH, Wall MJ Jr, Pepe PE, et al. Immediate versus delayed fluid resuscitation for hypotensive patients with penetrating torso injuries. N Engl J Med 1994; 331(17):1105–9.

37. Cotton BA, Jerome R, Collier BR, et al. Guidelines for prehospital fluid resuscitation in the injured patient. J Trauma 2009;67(2):389–402.

38. Sharpnack DD, Phillips YY. The pathology of primary blast injury. In: Zajtchuk R, Bellamy RF, Quick CM, editors. Conventional warfare: Ballistic, blast and burn injuries. Washington, DC: Office of the Surgeon General; 1992. p. 271–94.

39. Avidan V, Hersch M, Armon Y, et al. Blast lung injury: clinical manifestations, treatment, and outcome. Am J Surg 2005;190(6):927–31.

40. Aboudara M, Mahoney PF, Hicks B, et al. Primary blast lung injury at a NATO role 3 hospital. J R Army Med Corps 2014;160(2):161–6.

41. Sorkine P, Szold O, Kluger Y, et al. Permissive hypercapnia ventilation in patients with severe pulmonary blast injury. J Trauma 1998;45(1):35–8.

42. Ficke JR, Eastridge BJ, Butler FK, et al. Dismounted complex blast injury report of the army dismounted complex blast injury task force. J Trauma Acute Care Surg 2012;73:S520–34.

43. Bulger EM, Snyder D, Schoelles K, et al. An evidence-based prehospital guideline for external hemorrhage control: American College of Surgeons Committee on Trauma. Prehosp Emerg Care 2014;18(2):163–73.

44. Kragh JF Jr, Walters TJ, Baer DG, et al. Practical use of emergency tourniquets to stop bleeding in major limb trauma. J Trauma 2008;64(2 Suppl):S38–49 [discussion: S49–50].

45. Beekley AC, Sebesta JA, Blackbourne LH, et al. Prehospital tourniquet use in Operation Iraqi Freedom: effect on hemorrhage control and outcomes. J Trauma 2008;64(2 Suppl):S28–37 [discussion: S37].

46. Bumbasirevic M, Lesic A, Mitkovic M, et al. Treatment of blast injuries of the extremity. J Am Acad Orthop Surg 2006;14(10 Spec No):S77–81.

47. Lin DL, Kirk KL, Murphy KP, et al. Orthopedic injuries during Operation Enduring Freedom. Mil Med 2004;169(10):807–9.

48. Langworthy MJ, Smith JM, Gould M. Treatment of the mangled lower extremity after a terrorist blast injury. Clin Orthop Relat Res 2004;(422):88–96.

49. DePalma RG, Burris DG, Champion HR, et al. Blast injuries. N Engl J Med 2005; 352(13):1335–42.

50. Ritenour AE, Baskin TW. Primary blast injury: update on diagnosis and treatment. Crit Care Med 2008;36(7 Suppl):S311–7.

51. Rosenfeld JV, McFarlane AC, Bragge P, et al. Blast-related traumatic brain injury. Lancet Neurol 2013;12(9):882–93.

52. Magnuson J, Leonessa F, Ling GS. Neuropathology of explosive blast traumatic brain injury. Curr Neurol Neurosci Rep 2012;12(5):570–9.

53. Snell FI, Halter MJ. A signature wound of war: mild traumatic brain injury. J Psychosoc Nurs Ment Health Serv 2010;48(2):22–8.

54. Hicks RR, Fertig SJ, Desrocher RE, et al. Neurological effects of blast injury. J Trauma 2010;68(5):1257–63.

55. Mac Donald CL, Johnson AM, Cooper D, et al. Detection of blast-related traumatic brain injury in U.S. military personnel. N Engl J Med 2011;364(22): 2091–100.

56. Carlson KF, Kehle SM, Meis LA, et al. Prevalence, assessment, and treatment of mild traumatic brain injury and posttraumatic stress disorder: a systematic review of the evidence. J Head Trauma Rehabil 2011;26(2):103–15.

57. Luoto TM, Silverberg ND, Kataja A, et al. Sport concussion assessment tool 2 in a civilian trauma sample with mild traumatic brain injury. J Neurotrauma 2014;31(8): 728–38.

58. Cole WR, Arrieux JP, Schwab K, et al. Test-retest reliability of four computerized neurocognitive assessment tools in an active duty military population. Arch Clin Neuropsychol 2013;28(7):732–42.

59. Bogdanova Y, Verfaellie M. Cognitive sequelae of blast-induced traumatic brain injury: recovery and rehabilitation. Neuropsychol Rev 2012;22(1): 4–20.

60. Sample PL, Greene D, Johns NR. Life-bombing-injury-life: a qualitative follow-up study of Oklahoma City bombing survivors with TBI. Brain Inj 2012;26(13–14): 1670–83.

61. Eikermann M, Velmahos G, Abbara S, et al. Case records of the Massachusetts General Hospital. Case 11-2014. A man with traumatic injuries after a bomb explosion at the Boston Marathon. N Engl J Med 2014;370(15):1441–51.

62. Luria S, Rivkin G, Avitzour M, et al. Comparative outcome of bomb explosion injuries versus high-powered gunshot injuries of the upper extremity in a civilian setting. Isr Med Assoc J 2013;15(3):148–52.
63. Saltychev M, Eskola M, Tenovuo O, et al. Return to work after traumatic brain injury: systematic review. Brain Inj 2013;27(13–14):1516–27.
64. Nichol AD, Higgins AM, Gabbe BJ, et al. Measuring functional and quality of life outcomes following major head injury: common scales and checklists. Injury 2011;42(3):281–7.
65. Cancelliere C, Kristman VL, Cassidy JD, et al. Systematic review of return to work after mild traumatic brain injury: results of the International Collaboration on Mild Traumatic Brain Injury Prognosis. Arch Phys Med Rehabil 2014;95(3 Suppl): S201–9.
66. Carroll LJ, Cassidy JD, Cancelliere C, et al. Systematic review of the prognosis after mild traumatic brain injury in adults: cognitive, psychiatric, and mortality outcomes: results of the International Collaboration on Mild Traumatic Brain Injury Prognosis. Arch Phys Med Rehabil 2014;95(3 Suppl):S152–73.
67. Rauh MJ, Aralis HJ, Melcer T, et al. Effect of traumatic brain injury among U.S. servicemembers with amputation. J Rehabil Res Dev 2013;50(2):161–72.
68. Lannin NA, Laver K, Henry K, et al. Effects of case management after brain injury: a systematic review. NeuroRehabilitation 2014;35(4):635–41.
69. Perla LY, Jackson PD, Hopkins SL, et al. Transitioning home: comprehensive case management for America's heroes. Rehabil Nurs 2013;38(5):231–9.

Printed and bound by CPI Group (UK) Ltd, Croydon, CR0 4YY

03/10/2024

01040488-0012